LIFE WISH

❀ LIFE WISH ❀

JILL IRELAND

LITTLE, BROWN AND COMPANY
Boston   Toronto

FIRST EDITION

The author is grateful to the following for permission to use
copyrighted material:

"HELLO & GOODBYE" Music by Elmer Bernstein, Words by
Alan & Marilyn Bergman, from the motion picture, FROM
NOON TILL THREE. © 1976 UNITED ARTISTS CORPORATION.
Rights Assigned to CBS CATALOGUE PARTNERSHIP. All Rights
Controlled & Administered by CBS UNART CATALOG INC. and
CBS CATALOG INC. All Rights Reserved. International Copy-
right Secured. Used by permission.

Excerpt from *Getting Well Again* by O. Carl Simonton, M.D.,
Stephanie Matthews-Simonton, and James L. Creighton. Copy-
right © 1978 by O. Carl Simonton and Stephanie Matthews-
Simonton. Reprinted by permission of Bantam Books, Inc. All
rights reserved.

Library of Congress Cataloging-in-Publication Data

Ireland, Jill.
Life wish.

1. Ireland, Jill—Health. 2. Breast—Cancer—
Patients—United States—Biography. I. Title.
RC280.B8I64 1987   362.1'9699449'00924 [B]   86-27768
ISBN 0-316-10926-6

Published simultaneously in Canada
by Little, Brown & Company (Canada) Limited

PRINTED IN THE UNITED STATES OF AMERICA

To my family

ACKNOWLEDGMENTS

WHEN I WAS TOLD I had cancer, I would have loved to talk to someone who had had the disease. I had watched several people close to me suffer from cancer, but unhappily none of them survived. It helped me through my initial terror that Happy Rockefeller and Betty Ford had overcome breast cancer; they were walking around now smiling and healthy, weren't they? I clung to this: if they could do it, so could I.

I am grateful to those two women for being publicly candid about their personal battles with cancer. It made a difference to me. With this in mind, I started this book as a companion for anyone unfortunate enough to be going through the isolation of catastrophic illness.

I intended the book to be helpful to others, but it soon became my companion, a means of self-discovery and personal growth. For seven months it seemed to write itself. Each day I awoke and was able to cast off the miasma of being a cancer victim with the knowledge that awaiting me downstairs along with my morning cup of tea was a brand-new yellow legal pad and a clear plastic Ziploc bag filled with a multitude of brightly colored felt-tipped pens.

There are many debts of gratitude that I would like to acknowledge, special people I am compelled to thank, starting with my doctors:

Alexander Culiner, Raymond Weston, Mitchell Karlan, Robert Uyeda and Michael Van Scoy Mosher. I am indebted to them not only for their medical and psychological expertise but for their warmth, affection and humor, all of which were as comforting to me as their ministrations were healing.

My holistic therapists, Dr. O. Carl Simonton, Sue Colin and Bernard Dowson.

My brother, John, and sister-in-law Sandra Ireland, who were the first to read my initial one hundred pages and urged me to continue. Cheerfully, Sandra offered to type subsequent pages, which she did patiently and uncomplainingly for nine months.

Sue Overholt, my secretary and possibly the only other person in the world who can interpret my longhand, typed day and night, keeping her sense of humor through painful bouts of rewriteitis.

King Zimmerman and Susie Dotan, whose friendship and support were invaluable. Marcia Borie for her initial suggestion that I write this book.

Michael Viner, my manager, who one cold snowy February day in Vermont read my book, liked it and introduced me to my agent, Mort Janklow.

Vernon Scott, whose friendship, faith and confidence helped me transform those first five hundred unruly pages into this book.

My editor, Fredrica S. Friedman, of Little, Brown, for her counsel and wisdom.

A special and profound debt of gratitude must be paid my dear friend Alan Marshall, who lived each page of this manuscript with me, contributing loving encouragement every step of the way.

Finally, thank you, Charlie, Suzanne, Paul, Tony, Jason, Valentine, Katrina and Zuleika. I love you.

Jill Ireland

LIFE WISH

1

Malignant!
Insidious, ugly, horrifying word. It slammed across the room at me, with almost physical force.

I had just undergone a biopsy. I was sick, giddy and disoriented; but as I was wheeled back into my room, I managed to ask my husband, "Did you see my doctor?"

"Yes."

"What did he say?"

The reply was spoken simply. "It's malignant. You are having a mastectomy tomorrow."

Cancer! I felt a flame of fear deep in my gut.

"Why didn't they operate while I was out? Why didn't they? No. I won't. I can't go through that again." I pushed away the plastic vomit dish. "I can't face the anesthetic. I can't go through the post-operating room again. Oh, why didn't they do it while I was out? Why?"

The outburst brought another attack of the awful nausea. God, this was a nightmare.

"Why didn't they take it while I was out?" Now I was angry. My right breast was burning with pain. All I could think was that I would have to face this again tomorrow. I managed to cry and vomit at the same time.

Charlie looked at me, shattered. I'd never seen an expression like it in his eyes before. "I tried to get them to do it, but they said they had to wake you and tell you. . . ."

In those first moments the impact of the consequences of cancer had not entered my mind. All I could handle was my immediate pain. It was a step down a road that would have no end. Now I know you don't get over cancer. Hopefully, you outlive it. But as I lay there recovering from a biopsy performed under general anesthetic that June 1, 1984, I had a great deal to learn, many battles to be fought.

Married to the man I loved, a mother to seven children, I was leading a full and happy life. With one slash of a surgeon's knife, everything was imperiled. My God, my daughter was only twelve years old. I was filled with horror. This couldn't be happening.

It wasn't until many months after Charlie spoke those terrifying words in the hospital that I determined to discover, if I could, why me?

This, then, is my moment of truth.

2

I WAS THE FIRSTBORN of John and Dorothy Ireland. They named me Jill Dorothy. We lived on a pretty, tree-lined street in a suburb of London with my baby brother, John. Each house was red brick with a flower-filled front garden surrounded by a well-trimmed privet hedge. My parents' house had a blue front door on which the name *Chertsy* was inscribed. I didn't know then and I don't know to this day what the name meant. But to me it made our house special.

I thought my father was very handsome, dark-haired with golden skin, large brown eyes with long black lashes and perfect, even features. He had a ready wit, a good singing voice and a conversational flair. He was a popular man who liked to socialize. High on his priorities was his pint of beer with friends. He kept the front and back gardens immaculate; the roses and the lawn were his great pride.

My mother was blue-eyed, with fair skin and hair, a true Anglo-Saxon. As a young woman she had a very feminine figure, rounded and soft, not athletic. Her brain, however, was athletic. She had a sharp, often caustic wit and she was good at arithmetic, capable of working out large, complicated problems in her head in seconds. To my amazement, she also could juggle three oranges in one hand. My mother liked to laugh and knew how to enjoy the moment. She kept house impeccably, never allowing me or anyone else to help her, saying, "If you want somethng done properly, do it yourself."

My parents often went dancing and I loved to see them off for an evening, Mummy in a long, sparkling dress and Daddy so debonair in his suit or, on a big night, his dinner jacket. They were a passionate couple who lived, loved and fought with gusto.

My mother's father was a mounted policeman who came from three generations of horsemen and country landowners in Dorset. My mother's mother was reared on a large, successful dairy farm. My own father managed a chain of grocery stores. His father, my paternal grandfather, had been a coachman. And my father, as a boy, had worked in the livery stables. He loved horses. Can such traits be inherited? I suppose they can. In any event, I grew up with a great love of horses and riding.

But it was not horseback riding that occupied my childhood. I can still recapture an early memory. I was four years old, holding my mother's hand as we walked through the tree-lined suburban streets. Dry autumn leaves crunched under my feet as I hurried to keep up with her determined stride. That was a special day. I was happy to be going somewhere alone with Mummy, without my baby brother, John. We weren't just on a stroll; my mother was excited and full of purpose.

"But where are we going, Mummy?"

"You'll see." She was puffed up with the secret.

"But where?" I was excited now.

"You'll see when we get there."

We crossed a hardtop road and found ourselves at a churchlike building. We entered the building. And life began.

I heard a piano. I know now it was classical music, Delibes to be precise. Then, it was magic music to me. With a hollow, haunting sound, it echoed through the long corridors. We entered a room occupied by rows of small children wearing pale pink silk tunics tied at the waist with satin ribbons, their hair pulled back in satin bands. On their feet, shiny pink slippers — I had never seen anything like it. A dark-haired

6

woman stopped the music with a wave of her hand and approached us. I no longer remember the conversation she held with my mother. I only recall dancing in my socks with the other children to the beautiful music.

My mother sat on a wooden chair along a wall with the other "Mummies." She looked happy as I made my first attempt at a balletic leap, a grand jeté. I was enrolled in the Stella Mainwering School of Ballet, Tap and Elocution.

I remember the ballet, acrobatic and tap classes. I remember my first solo in one of many recitals. I danced to the music of *Coppélia*: *Da Da DAA-DA Da DAA-DA De Dudaly DA DA DA*. I can still dance the first steps. I remember my pink satin shoes and the cotton wrapped around my toes, sticking to the blisters as I peeled it off. I remember the many ballet exams and my copy of *First Steps* by William Franch, the small ballet dancer's bible. I remember the happy times. According to my inordinately proud mother, I danced with such talent and ability on my first visit that Miss Stella, as we called her, asked if I had taken lessons.

I remained happily with Miss Stella until she married and moved to a far-off land called America. Then I was taken to Gladys Harmer's dancing school, a more pressurized environment. I was ten, old enough to make the trip alone on a bus. I was not as happy as I had been at Miss Stella's. When, I wonder, did the happiness stop and a sense of responsibility, an obsession to succeed, take over? When did I lose my chance to choose? The other girls were competitive. They were good, extraordinarily good. One was expected to win medals at the prestigious all-England dance festivals. One was also required to receive honors in the endless ballet examinations given in French by licensed examiners. They were a source of constant worry and pressure. I developed a nervous sniffing, even when I slept. Sniff, sniff, sniff.

"Jill, stop sniffing," my mother would call through the wall.

Next step up the ladder was a professional child's dancing and acting school, the Corona Academy in Chiswick, London.

Now I rode the bus and a train to the high-powered school that provided children for movies and the theater. Several child stars attended the school. My father hardly seemed to figure in my life. My mother, energetic, vital and determined, prevailed. She urged, cajoled and encouraged me. She told me much later it had given her a social outlet, a means of self-expression. Once a week she bought a copy of the *Stage* and scoured it for child auditions. By the time I was twelve, I had appeared in pantomime, and danced in the children's ballet as one of the fairies in *Cinderella*. Once a week I was allowed to leave school early to play in Thursday matinees.

At fourteen, I joined the *3 J's* — Jean, Jeanette and Jill. We danced, sang and performed acrobatics at balls, Masonic dinners and occasional church socials. Then at fifteen and a half I became a Tiller Girl, a sort of Rockette, at the London Palladium. This necessitated an hour-long journey with a forty-five-minute walk to and from the station. Frightened and alone well after midnight, I walked the center of the road. It was dark, silent and quite terrifying. At last I would see my house. Key in shaking hand, I would open the door and creep upstairs to bed to sniff myself to sleep. That was my routine every night for five months. When the Palladium job ended I danced in the musical *Wish You Were Here,* then another, *Wonderful Time.* I was sixteen when my parents gave me permission to share a London apartment with a girlfriend. I was happily relieved of my midnight runs.

At seventeen I spent springtime in Paris, dancing with the Anita Avila Ballet Company. Later that summer I danced in Monte Carlo's Sporting Club. The highlight of that season was an invitation to Prince Rainier's annual Red Cross Ball, a black-tie affair. None of the ballet dancers owned an evening gown, although some had cocktail dresses. All I had was the taffeta skirt I wore with a strapless bathing suit for a bodice. I clipped earrings to my shoes to make them look like evening slippers, and off I went. It was a wonderful experience, my first sight of real luxury, of wealthy men and stunning women.

When I was eighteen I appeared in the movie *Oh, Rosalinda,* dancing a solo role. My performance attracted the J. Arthur Rank Organization, whch signed me to a film contract. By the time I was twenty I had starred in several movies. A year later I married a handsome young actor, David McCallum, and thirteen months later I became the mother of a son, Paul. I don't remember making conscious decisions to do all this. It just happened.

While I was pregnant, the Rank Organization suspended my contract. Suspecting they would, I had concealed my condition until I couldn't fit into a champagne silk evening gown "the Organization" had especially designed for me to wear to premieres and balls. David and I were to attend a premiere at the Odeon Theatre in Leicester Square as one of our contractual obligations. The limousine arrived promptly, early enough to give me time to get into my finery. There were the evening gown and fur waiting on the backseat of the limo. The Rank Organization, never philanthropic, kept my dress-up clothes in the studio wardrobe department, delivering them just for the occasion. When I returned home after the ball or other events, I removed my fancy clothes and the driver put them back in the limousine; then like a rather large pumpkin, it drove off, leaving me clad in an old terry-cloth robe. This time, horrors, the dress refused to zip up. David tried. I tried. No good. What now? I couldn't *not* turn up. I'd played truant too often. There was no choice; I had to wear a dress of my own. It would surely cause trouble and end in harsh comments from Rank's higher echelons. But it seemed the best solution under the circumstances. I didn't own many clothes. I tended to look like a beatnik in my civvies: black slacks, black shirt and leather thong sandals. Standing before my closet in my underwear, I frantically slid my few things along the rod. I had recently bought a plain gray silk dress from Fenwicks in Bond Street, attracted by its modest price. It was simple and suitable to my age, not at all glamorous and sexy like the creation I had failed to zip. The Organization insisted on a certain image for its contract players. We were members of what they called the Rank Charm School. We were supposed to be well-bred, society-type girls who acted for fun. We wore elegant gowns provided by the studio. My gray dress didn't fit the portrait, but I wore it. David, who was desperate because his own contract was threatened by this whole affair, said I looked nice. I draped the rented fur over my shoulders and off we went. I encountered a sea of raised eyebrows. The following day I was questioned. I confessed, and my movie contract was suspended.

If Mr. Rank did not want his swelling actress, many other studios and theater productions did. During my pregnancy I appeared on stage at night and worked at movie studios in the day. In *The Diary of Anne Frank* I mastered the art of walking sideways while still facing the audience. I looked pregnant only from the side view, so I moved, sat and spoke with my body facing out front. I played Margot, Anne Frank's sickly sister. The script required the cast to remain onstage throughout the play. Margot spent much of the time resting on a couch. I'm afraid Margot, and Jill, fell asleep more than once.

After Paul's birth, the Organization measured my waist to certify I had returned to my prepregnant eighteen inches. I had. My contract was renewed for another year. Looking back, I remember working, going to class and keeping in shape. I was ready for any job that might come up. I took care of my clothes; actresses need to dress well. I took care of my shoes; actresses need good shoes. I saved my money — you never knew when you would be out of work. I took care of my figure, hair and skin. And finally I controlled my sniff. David was much in demand as an actor. Both of us worked regularly; we were considered a successful young couple. Sophisticates, we thought ourselves, juggling our work, marriage and parenthood. I loved acting in spite of never feeling I was good enough, never feeling satisfied with my performances.

Then still in my twenties, as Miss Stella had done eighteen years earlier, we moved to the far-off land, America.

3

I WAS AT HOME, lying naked under a towel on the massage table in my dressing room, divorced, remarried — many movies, countries and children later. My masseuse, a small, dark-haired Russian named Jana, worked on my body as we talked and gossiped about things women discuss when they're alone in their private world, concerned only for that moment with the preservation of beauty. Jana massaged my thighs with strong, kneading fingers. Her purpose was to make sure not one bubble of cellulite would mar the line of my legs.

Massages were new for me. I'd started them four weeks earlier in a desperate attempt to get back into shape after the most recent of a series of leg injuries. My right leg had atrophied; the muscle tone was weak. I'd been exercising, but that wasn't enough. I had been advised that massage was good for the circulation. Jana was a cosmetic masseuse, dedicated to keeping women's bodies flawless. Wonderful! I was getting therapeutic massage and my thighs were looking swell. I wanted my legs to look good again for myself and for my husband, Charlie.

Charlie . . . I thought of him while Jana worked away. I fell in love with Charles Bronson in Bavaria during the filming of *The Great Escape* in 1962, shortly after I'd suffered a miscarriage. I'd just come out of the hospital and was on my first outing when I was introduced to Charlie, along with other members of the cast and crew, at the rushes of the previous week's work. It was pouring rain afterward and I made a run for the car, where David waited behind the wheel. I would have been soaked to the skin had not Charlie come to my rescue with an umbrella. As I got into the car he gave me a boyish grin that seemed, even on such short acquaintance, to be appealingly out of character.

I couldn't help being physically attracted to him. He was thirty-nine years old and he was gorgeous. It was obviously mutual, although both of us were married. It was his eyes, his fantastic body, that longish dark hair and his attitude of confidence in the way he stood. He was different from any man I'd ever known, almost broodingly quiet and intense, with an explosive air of violence about him. It seemed I was also something different for Mr. Bronson. So as opposites often attract, the inevitable happened. It was love at first sight for both of us.

The ninth child and the seventh son, Charlie was born of Lithuanian parents, Walter and Mary Buchinsky, in the small Pennsylvania mining town of Ehrenfeld (known locally as Scooptown). His grandmother ran a boardinghouse for Russian immigrants. It was in this house that Mary Valinksy met Walter Buchinsky. She was fourteen years old the day she was awakened by her mother with the command to get up and get dressed. "Today you are getting married." Of course this dialogue took place in Lithuanian. The child began to cry.

"I don't want to get married. Who am I going to marry?"

Little Mary hid under her bed, cowering close to the wall, while her mother extricated her with a long-handled broom, announcing that her future husband was to be Walter, one of the many boarders who were staying in the house.

She was married that day.

Mary had a beautiful singing voice and was a member of the church choir. All of her children were reared as Catholics. It was a hard life, made more so when Walter died in his early forties, leaving Mary alone with her responsibilities. Charlie's early life was full of deprivation. It made him in many ways a tough, withdrawn child. His nickname as a boy was "Shulty," Russian for cold. His best friend was his dog, Duke.

At the time I met Charlie, I felt guilty about everything in my life. David and I had moved to Los Angeles. We had two more children, Jason and Valentine, each child giving me another reason to continue with my marriage until I had the courage to face divorce. I was ill a great deal of the time. I was getting a divorce and I was stressed out. I was a working mother at a time when it was unfashionable, accompanied by guilt over leaving my children to work five days a week in a TV series titled "Shane," co-starring David Carradine. I felt guilty about divorce, guilty about working when my three sons needed me, guilty about my affair with a married man. All I felt was guilt.

Finally, my immune system broke down. I became desperately ill with a strep throat. The doctor gave me Rondomycin, to which I had a severe allergic reaction. I was deeply anxious, so he gave me a tranquilizing shot for the anxiety. He didn't realize, however, that my illness was compounded by the allergic reaction to the medicine he was already giving me. I became more and more ill. My face, hands and legs were swollen and I ran a fever almost constantly. I had trouble breathing and shook all over.

A friend, Marcia Borie, sang the praises of Dr. Raymond Weston. She said, "He's a genius, Jill, a wonderful human being and a great diagnostician." So Ray Weston entered my life. He immediately recognized my allergic reaction and gave me a shot of ACTH. He took over my health care from that day on. He was always there for me, which was good, as I was constantly ill — low blood pressure, severe allergic reactions, rheumatism, phlebitis, flu, sore throats, thyroid condition, broken kneecap, broken tibia, torn ligaments, bad rashes and back injuries.

David and I were divorced in 1967. Charlie and I were married in 1968. My health improved. We had custody of my three boys, Paul, Jason and Valentine, along with Charlie's two children, Suzanne and Tony. It took a domicile the size of our large Bel Air house to blend the two families. We had our problems, but I was determined to be perfect in my role of wife and mother, as well as stepmother. And perfect in my role of actress.

During the early years of our marriage Charlie and I worked in many films together. Among them, *Violent City, Cold Sweat, Someone Behind the Door, Breakout, Hard Times.* For about four years, from 1969 to 1973, we traveled Europe making movies, three a year during our busiest period. We always took the children, ranging in age from five to thirteen years, and the pets with us — a traveling circus. Two actors, five children, three dogs and a cat and a partridge in a pear tree. We traveled to London, Paris, the south of France, Rome and Istanbul — all in one year! It was fun, exciting and hectic, and probably stressful, but I think I blew off the stress when I acted. I loved acting. It provided a release valve. Also, Charlie and I were very much in love. Our relationship was a passionate, stormy, loving festival of emotions at all times. That also blew off a lot of steam. In any event, I survived with very few illnesses, perhaps only one a year, which was good for me.

Although motion pictures have provided a fine living, it is nevertheless a strange occupation for Charles Bronson. He doesn't enjoy being photographed. In fact, I tell him that he's like the Indian who, when his photograph was taken, thought a piece of his soul had been stolen. Charlie should know better. His soul is inviolate, belonging completely to him.

Charlie is a man of few words, a man who can sit in comfortable silence while people around him chatter, trying to know him. Charlie never seeks company. He has little patience with the rounds of social engagements and attendant publicity. It is out of character. His nature is suited to the woods, to the quiet of nature. He is a true loner, a male animal in every sense of the word. He is, though, a family man. His friends are his children. His social life begins at seven o'clock when we all sit down for dinner. By 1971, we were also the parents of Zuleika.

Zuleika. Ah! Zuleika. Named after writer Max Beerbohm's

scandalous heroine, Zuleika Dobson, my daughter was conceived in Paris, carried in Spain, shipped through London and delivered in Los Angeles. She is the only child Charlie and I have together, the apple of her father's eye and my most precious treasure. My daughter, oh the pleasure she gives us.

Zuleika is as strongly independent as her parents, but very much her own person, possessed of proud carriage and quiet dignity. One minute she is the picture of Charlie, the next I see a younger me. Tall for her age, Zuleika speaks slowly and with an almost aristocratic grace and cadence — and God knows where she gets that. She's an athlete and a serious horsewoman. Her bookshelves are lined with trophies, silver trays, dishes and medals, bedecked with blue ribbons won in national horse shows where Zuleika has been embarrassed by public-address systems blaring: "Now on deck, Tudor's Dillon, owned by Zuleika Farm, ridden by Zuleika Bronson."

She has threatened to change her name to Sandy.

My man of few words had had a thing or two to say on the subject of what he called "women's clutter." He complained that when he washed his face in our bathroom, his elbows knocked over lotion bottles. There were expletives as he became entangled in negligees hanging behind the door when he tried to extricate his robe from layers of chiffon. Showers were a problem, too. Exasperated, he would move my underwear from the shower door, where I liked to hang lingerie after rinsing. He never knew where to put all the small, awkward-to-handle bikini panties, lacy bras and flimsy tights that slid mockingly to the floor whenever he tried to hang them carefully on the towel racks. Charlie finally proclaimed he did not want women's things around the bedroom and bath. So, banished, I converted an adjoining room into a dressing room.

I love it. A female sanctuary, a room of my own, it is lined with mirrors. Every wall is a closet with mirrored doors. An antique four-poster bed, which once rested in my home in England, now stands between two French doors, which lead to a veranda overlooking the Bel Air golf course. Over the fireplace two nineteenth-century pastel paintings seem perfectly at home. A large, rose velvet armchair and footrest sit to the left of the fireplace near the Chippendale desk, which also once had been in residence in England. Beside a window is an ornately carved antique oak dressing table surrounded with theatrical lights. The effect is practical and attractive. I keep all my feminine "women's things," as Charlie calls them, in this room. It is also my cat's bedroom. Polar, my blue point Siamese, considers it *our* room. She sleeps there alone at night. I use it during the day.

My room always has the light scent of my favorite perfume. The walls are covered in fabric adorned with bunches of lilac and pink blossoms; the same material is used in the draperies surrounding the four-poster. The windows are curtained in a pale pink, shot silk taffeta. There is a Persian rug on the highly polished parquet floor. It is a beautiful room, entirely feminine, and it contains my personal treasures. There are three shelves of family pictures — my children's treasured baby portraits, pictures of my parents, sentimental photographs of my husband and myself, and pictures of favorite dogs, cats and horses. All are framed in antique silver and surrounded by mementos: my son Paul's baby rattle, daughter Zuleika's first mug with teeth marks on it, a small china box filled with seashells.

That day I watched myself in the mirror as Jana massaged. I looked pretty good, I thought. In my forties, I was planning a brave approach to fifty. I always planned and schemed in this room, campaigning to keep my thighs tight and my breasts firm. I exercised, massaged and clothed myself to become as ideal a me as I could be. According to Jana, if you had enough massages your body would stay young almost indefinitely.

I looked at my body, or at least what I could see of it from under the towel. Yes, it looked good. The breasts were firm and youthful, the stomach taut, the thighs looked pretty damned good, thanks to massage and my four-mile daily run. The nose was a bit long. I wished I had the courage to shorten it, but the thought of surgery scared me. I hoped never to have any. The hair — thick, one of my better features. Some gray was coming in around the temples, but it really wasn't noticeable, as it blended in with the blond and made highlights. I never spent time at the hairdresser. My hair really was "wash and wear." In fact, my three hours of massage with Jana every week was my biggest investment in beauty for the future.

4

 I WAS SHAKEN from my reverie by the telephone. "Hello."

It was my eldest, Paul, speaking in a voice I had never heard before.

"Hello, Mom. I'm in terrible pain. I'm in more pain than I've ever been in my life. I feel terrible."

"Where are you, Paul?"

There were gasps as he pulled himself together. "I'm with my friend Henry at the emergency room at Cedars-Sinai. Oh, I feel terrible, Mom. I'm in terrible pain."

I paid Jana, who left, saying she hoped Paul was all right. I quickly slipped on shorts, a man's shirt and tennis shoes. I ran to the master bedroom, where Charlie was watching the evening news.

He looked up, startled, immediately picking up on my concern. "What's wrong, babe?"

"Charlie, Paul just called." As I spoke, the phone rang again and I grabbed it. This time it was Paul's friend Henry.

"Hello, Jill. Paul's here with me. My father's a doctor and he's checking Paul right now. He thinks Paul is having a kidney stone attack."

"Henry, thank you very much. Have you called our family physician? Please call Doctor Raymond Weston," and I gave him the telephone number. I trusted Ray completely and wanted him there for Paul.

I went to the hospital while Charlie stayed at home with Zuleika and our adoptive daughter, Katrina, sixteen. Ray Weston was at Paul's side.

"They've given him a lot of morphine, dear. It's a kidney stone. We're hoping he will pass it."

After an agonizing night, he did. Paul recovered, but it was a trauma for me. During the previous eighteen months, I had gone through many traumas. My father had had a heart attack, open-heart surgery and a subsequent stroke. My friend Hilary Holden died suddenly, and Charlie and I had taken into our home her daughter, Katrina. Katrina and my daughter became close. Zuleika enjoyed having a sister near her in age. A basically happy girl, Katrina did well in our family. However, blending a new personality into our life did mean more activities and responsibilities. This also took its toll on my health. One day while hosing down the dog run I slipped and fell, tearing all the ligaments in my lower right leg, which resulted in three months on crutches. Then I had a riding accident in which I broke my leg, requiring ten more months on crutches. So I had been dragging around in casts and metal braces using walking sticks for nearly two years.

It was during this time that my brother entered the hospital in Toronto for extensive tests and received good news and bad news. The good news was that his tumor was not a glomus jugulare and required no surgery for the time being. The bad news was that he suffered a venous malformation, a trapped blood vessel, rather like a bubble in an inner tube and inoperable, possibly congenital. Also during this incredible year Charlie's brother Joe died in a Los Angeles hospital as he awaited surgery. We had given a dinner party for Joe just the week before and he had been so happy. His death was sad and a sudden blow.

Now I was recovering, finally, from two consecutive breaks of my left leg. The most recent was a ten-month-long injury suffered when one of my horses fell on me. Horses play a major role in my life. They are my means of mixing business with pleasure. Horses are beautiful, powerful, sensitive animals, exhilarating to ride and show. And sometimes they can be a profitable enterprise.

Charlie and I established Zuleika Farm East in Vermont many years ago, indulging both Charlie's love of solitude and my love of horseflesh. Having spent many years riding in movies, these days Charlie's interest in the animals is mostly as a spectator. His stable is full of motorbikes.

At this writing Zuleika Farm East has seven employees and twenty horses, not including boarders, at its training facilities, a brood mare program and four yearlings as well as several newborn babies. Boasting a large hunter-jumper ring, an indoor ring and a small jumper ring, an outdoor exercise track with two dressage rings and a complete cross-country course, it is perhaps the best equestrian facility in the area. Zuleika Farm West owns eight horses and boards an additional five under the management of three employees. The western establishment rests at the foot of the Malibu mountains in cozy little stables with banks of wild flowers bordering the riding rings and sandy roads.

It was in that innocent setting that one of my horses, Stutz Bearcat, and I met disaster. One night, almost a year before my fateful biopsy, I had finished working Stutz but thought I'd jump one more fence. I picked up a canter, rocked his weight back onto his haunches and approached the fence. It was a perfect approach, a perfect takeoff, and a calamitous landing. At the peak of the jump, he forgot to unfold his legs. Having no landing gear, he crashed to the ground. Poor Stutz. He frightened himself almost as much as he terrified me. He fell on his face, then rolled sideways onto my body. I remember going down, down, down, as if in slow motion, then tipping over, this huge animal falling on top of me. I realized if he didn't get off immediately, he could crush my pelvis, my ribs, maybe even kill me. I yelled, "Stutz, get up, Stutz!" He gained his feet but my foot caught in the stirrup; I couldn't extract it. He gave a yank, causing excruciating pain on top of what I already felt. I lay on the ground in a symphony of agony. Stutz was standing close by, trembling. Someone came to my side.

"Come on, Bronson, you're all right."

"No," I said quietly, "I'm not all right. I'm hurt."

From various past injuries I knew by the degree of pain this was serious.

I spoke so quietly nobody really thought I was in major trouble. I was helped to the bench, then left alone. Someone put my horse back in his stall. I sat for a long time before Pesty, a junior rider and family friend, telephoned Charlie, who took me to see a bone specialist. He had gone home, so I was treated by his associate. My leg was braced between two sticks and taped. I was given crutches and some codeine and sent home. I spent the most painful night of my life.

The next morning, tired and nauseated from the codeine and nonstop agony, I was taken to see the bone specialist, who set the spiral fracture and put me in plaster. What a relief to have the bone realigned. How soothing and reassuring the warm plaster. I wore the cast for three and a half months. When it was removed my leg hadn't mended. On went the cast for another four months. This time the plaster didn't feel so soothing — or reassuring. Once again the leg failed to mend. I wore a cast for yet an additional three months. Then something new was introduced, EMI, Electromagnetic Impulse, a device that sent an electrical current through my injury. I wore the device ten hours a day for the final three months. I had torn every ligament in my lower right leg a year earlier, so I had been dragging around in casts and metal braces and using walking sticks for nearly two years.

Now, free from all that at last, I was thoroughly enjoying the feeling of fitness. My sense of well-being was enhanced by our return from a two-week Hawaiian vacation. While there, I started back on an exercising and eating-well regime. I began walking briskly two miles a day; and before our stay in Hawaii came to an end, Charlie and I pushed our walks to four miles, each mile taking about fourteen minutes. We returned to our Bel Air home suntanned, exercised and feeling good. I looked and felt better than I had in two years.

5

ON ONE PARTICULAR MAY Thursday in 1984, Charlie and I felt particularly energized, so we took off on a two-mile run. It was a beautiful day. On our return, happy and exhilarated from our exercise, we made love; then we showered and dressed ourselves and went out to lunch.

After lunch I was scheduled to see Dr. Mitchell Karlan for a routine breast checkup. Every spring before leaving for Vermont, I run the gamut of doctor's appointments for all the routine examinations women should undergo every six months. Mitch's office is in a chic area of Beverly Hills and was crowded. We told the nurse we would return and then hotfooted it over to Neiman-Marcus, always a favorite store of mine, where Charlie and I spent a pleasant hour browsing. While I ate some dark chocolate purchased at the wonderful candy counter, I bought a brave yellow hat with a purple and green band, then munched happily while I watched Charlie buy a rather dashing boater. It was perfect for keeping the sun off his head at horse shows, just the right touch of incongruity. Most of the horse-show people wore cowboy hats. It was fun being us. We enjoyed the privileges — health, wealth and leisure, one another's company. We thought things were wonderful, perfect. We were very happy.

We returned to Dr. Karlan's office. The waiting room had thinned out. It wasn't long before I was inside one of the small examination rooms, naked to the waist and holding a small cotton towel modestly in front of my chest. Soon Mitch came in and after a few pleasantries and a casual joke, he began the examination. My smile covered a deep-rooted anxiety that probably most women feel when they are examined this way. My breasts were a vulnerable area. It wasn't uncommon for me to have the occasional lump. I suffered from mastitis for years and lived through the comings and goings of many swellings and small lumps. They had always been nothing to worry about. Today I told Mitch that I had been having a strange burning and tingling sensation in my right breast. Also I had a lump situated close to my armpit.

With his eyes closed, he carefully palpated my breasts, felt under my arms and around my throat. I held my breath as Mitch examined me.

Finally, he said, "Well, in my opinion — and you can get a second opinion — you need a biopsy. There is an irregularity in the breasts. The right one has a different feel from the left. I really believe you should have a biopsy on Monday. Let's get it over with."

I was surprised but not frightened. "Do I have to have it in a hospital?"

"Yes. It could be done in the office, but you should have a general anesthetic. I would like you to go upstairs to the X-ray department and have a mammogram taken. Your examination in November was normal, so let's see if there have been any changes in six months. Okay?"

"Okay," I said.

The radiologist's waiting room was familiar. I had been there many times before and I felt no apprehension when a nurse took me in for X rays. Once again, I stripped to the waist and both my breasts were lightly compressed beween the plates of the mammograph machine. I took the X rays back to Mitch and waited with Charlie. We were the last people in the waiting room, and after five minutes we saw one of the nurses leave for the day.

"Hmm, I should have stayed in Neiman-Marcus," I joked. Charlie smiled and stifled a yawn. He was hungry and this whole thing was taking too much time.

We were sure after Mitch saw the X rays there would be no biopsy on Monday, not for me anyway. I was fit and trim and in good shape. I wished I hadn't bothered with the X rays.

"I want to get home before the traffic gets heavy," said Charlie.

Mitch appeared in the doorway of the reception room and I moved toward him.

"Oh, and bring Charlie," he said.

In his office the X rays were on display, clipped up with a light behind them. Mitch gave me a penetrating look.

"I told you I thought you needed a biopsy, but now I am telling you you definitely need a biopsy. And after what I see, I'm taking you in tonight. We have to do it tomorrow. Now, look at the X rays. See those little white starlike points?"

·I looked. I could see them.

"You have calcifications there. We have to get them out and find out what they are."

I was shocked. "Tonight? I have to go in tonight? Can't it be tomorrow?"

"Well, all right. You can come in tomorrow. Be at admitting at seven-thirty, bright and early."

Suddenly I was tired. It didn't seem real. We followed Mitch down the hallway to the receptionist's office. One of his nurses was still there. Mitch telephoned an anesthesiologist.

"I want Doctor Wender. With your allergy history, I want to get him for you. He's the best, Jill."

Things were moving fast now. The nurse gave me a form with instructions for people about to have surgery. Mitch said, "Nothing to eat after midnight, promise? Nothing by mouth after midnight."

"I promise."

"All right, Jill. Don't worry. I'll see you tomorrow. All you need now is a little luck," he said. And home we went.

The evening passed normally. Some of the children were home for dinner. I mentioned the biopsy. No one seemed unduly concerned, including me. I told everyone it was a commonplace precaution for women my age. I told stories and joked in my usual lighthearted way at the dinner table, but deep in my heart there was no question. I knew I had cancer. Then I went upstairs, showered and washed my hair, lingering longer than usual in my dressing room. The last thing I did before I went to bed was write a letter to Zuleika.

I chose a special sheet of notepaper with a watermark. When held up to the light there appeared a small child offering an apple to a white pony that resembled Zuleika's own much-loved pony, Cheeky.

The note included two happy-face figures, one large with its arms around a smaller one. It was a signature I used on all the notes I wrote to Zuleika. It represented us. I placed the letter in an envelope and sealed it, writing her name on the outside; on the flap I felt compelled to reach out to her one more time. I wrote, "Please don't be sad for too long. I would hate you to be sad." Then once again I drew a large, round happy-face with a big smile, and placed the envelope in my jewelry box and locked it.

This is what I wrote in the letter:

This is being written in haste, so please don't use my spelling or writing as an example.

Love you X X X, Love you X X X, Love you X X X.

My dearest little girl. If you are reading this, sadly I have had to leave you, at least here on this Earth. But, darling, I will *always* be with you. I love you so much I couldn't possibly leave you completely. You have given me more happiness than anything in my life, my little girl. Know you are loved. Live a happy life. Try not to be sad for too long. That would make me sad. Every birthday you should pick out a piece of my jewelry as a birthday present from me with love. The rest will all be yours in time.

Zuleika, have faith in yourself. You are strong, smart, a really nice person. I know you will make the right decisions about things all your life, so believe in you.

Bye, bye for now, Baba. I know one day we will be together again. I love you so much.

Mom X X X

In the morning we were awakened by our alarm and I wondered, why so early? I quickly remembered, and for the first time, I felt the stirrings of fear. I needed a glass of water.

I recalled the doctor's admonition about not taking anything by mouth. I asked Charlie, "Do you think the doctor meant water? I suppose so. It's taken by mouth."

"Well, I don't think so," Charlie said. "After all, your surgery's scheduled for three-thirty this afternoon. The water will have gone through by then. It's only water."

I agreed. Besides, by now my mouth was dry and I felt bilious. I drank a full tumbler of water and threw a toothbrush and a nearly finished tube of toothpaste into my purse. I wasn't going to be in the hospital long. I took a last-minute look at my dressing room. I went to my bed and picked up the little happy-faced rag doll that Zuleika had given me for my birthday the year before. I tucked her into my purse to keep me company and off we went for Cedars-Sinai.

Zuleika had been born there nearly thirteen years earlier; my father had undergone open-heart surgery there. Only the week before, Paul had been admitted overnight, so we knew the hospital well and made straight for the admitting office. There we encountered another couple, husband and wife. She was ashen and carried a bed pillow. I judged her to be my age. We said good morning. She told me she was Dr. Mitchell Karlan's patient, too, and that she had had a biopsy the week before. The pathology report taken from the frozen section had been negative, but after further examination, it came up positive. So she was there this morning to have a mastectomy. The pillow, she said, was because she found hospital pillows hard as rocks.

Our husbands chatted, at first casually and cheerfully, and

then tensely. The men seemed shocked and helpless sitting there; one man beside his wounded wife, who was facing even greater onslaught, the other trying to think positively — his wife could never have cancer, not her. The biopsy was just a routine precaution. But why did everyone keep saying, "Good luck"?

I recalled Mitch's last words when I left his office the previous evening, "All you need now is a little luck." I'd thought at the time it sounded unmedical and unscientific and rather scary personally. Somehow I flinched each time a well-meaning nurse or hospital orderly said it. Good luck. Good luck? Good luck. It mocked me. However, I told myself medical science is based on more than luck, isn't it? So I blocked out their good lucks and tried to sit out the day in the hospital room with Charlie.

The IV nurse, "There you are. All hooked up. The anesthesiologist will go into the same tube. Good luck."

And Ray Weston, my own doctor, "Don't worry. Think positively. Everything is going to be all right. You have the best surgeon. I'll be there. Good luck."

The day crept on. Finally, they came with the words I was to remember and dread, "They've come to take you."

They have? Oh, no.

"Can you move yourself onto the gurney?"

Of course I can.

"Lie down now, we're on our way." I was wheeled down the long corridors to the operating suite. How elegant it sounded. We stopped outside — me, the nurse, my husband, Paul and the transportation man. I tried to look into the operation suite through the windows in the door. It seemed innocent enough. Oh God, oh God, I don't believe this. They're opening the doors and wheeling me in. The transportation man said, "Good luck," and left. Charlie and my son were given green gowns so they could wait with me. I was lying in a smallish room occupied by Charlie, Paul and Mitch Karlan. He had arrived full of energy, all covered in green, and said a few encouraging words.

Everyone was cheerful and making little jokes. It was a bizarre atmosphere in which I was the central figure, except I seemed to have lost control of the scenario and my persona. Dr. Wender, the anesthesiologist, arrived, also capped, gowned and masked in green. He had nice eyes, blue, concerned and kind.

"I do all the old people and heart-problem patients," he told me. "Now, have you eaten anything for twenty-four hours?"

"No, I haven't. I had a glass of water at six this morning, Doctor. But no food."

Dr. Wender's eyes did not look so pleased. He worked out the number of hours since the water. Then he said, "I'm sorry. We're going to have to tube you. I can't risk having fluid come up and choke you during surgery. Don't worry about the water. With the tube in your stomach, there will be no danger of this. Remember, Jill, you're safer here than out on the street or at home."

I was not reassured. I was now very, very scared.

"I'm going to give you something to calm you down," he said, holding aloft a huge syringe and needle.

"Oh, don't. I'd hate that." But it was too late. He was injecting the contents into my IV tube.

"This may make you taste onions."

"Oh, no, I'd hate that." I said it again, but I was already tasting garlic and onion vapors in my throat. I *did* hate it. The sensation was followed by wooziness. Oh, God, I feel helpless. I hate it. I hate it.

"We're wheeling you in now. Say good-bye to Charlie and Paul. You'll see them when you come back."

6

I CAME AROUND IN THE post-operation room. It was hard to struggle up out of unconsciousness. My right breast burned. I thought to myself, "They've gone ahead and done a mastectomy. My breast is gone. It hurts so much."

I had trouble breathing. My lungs felt floppy, and there was a numbness in my legs. My own doctor, Ray Weston, came over to see me.

"Stop that huffing and puffing."

I knew what he meant. I was hyperventilating. Obediently, I stopped, but I was still sick. The nurses in post-op were efficient and businesslike.

"Take deep breaths, Jill."

With great difficulty I did. I had trouble talking. My mouth wouldn't work. No one could understand anything I said. I was in post-op for three hours, sick and giddy. Finally, after what seemed hours, they wheeled me to my room. As soon as the motion started my nausea increased. The nurse held a vomit dish by my head as we progressed down the corridor and into an elevator. It was rough and bumpy. My breast burned. We came out of the elevator on the eighth floor, where they paused to let me vomit. I finally arrived in my room. Sanctuary. I wanted to cry. Charlie and my three sons were waiting. I smiled at them and received a big, cheery hello from Paul, a confused, wounded look from middle son Jason, and a numb-eyed, blank smile from Valentine, my youngest. Charlie looked tired, or was it shattered? I felt another wave of nausea.

"Vomit dish, nurse, please!"

I was introduced to my night nurse. I was to have twenty-four-hour nurses. I was to be spoiled, pampered and cared for the way most eighth-floor patients were. It was the VIP floor, after all. I vomited and turned to meet my husband's eyes.

It was then Charlie told me the tumor was malignant, that I was to have a mastectomy the following day.

It was the worst thing I could have heard at that moment. More anesthetic, more surgery. I vomited more fluid and cried harder. I wasn't worried about losing my breast as much as I was truly terrified of the anesthetic and recovery room. It had been such a nightmare. My breast hurt so much after a simple biopsy, what would it be like regaining consciousness after they cut all of it off? I cried and cried. I wanted a way out. I couldn't see one. I would have to go through with it. Oh, God, I didn't believe any of this. I was inconsolable.

Charlie, tired with red-rimmed eyes, stroked my head and comforted me as best he could. I was grateful to him for telling me the truth from the start. Our relationship was based on honesty. There was no way he could lie to me as the doctors had requested.

"Wait until this evening," the doctors had urged him.

"I can't. She'll know as soon as she looks at me. I'll have to tell her the truth when she asks."

Charlie was right. I would have hated to be told something reassuring only to be given the truth later. This way I suffered the nausea and bad news all at once. And, in any case, there were those eyes. Those eyes could never lie to me.

It was eight hours after surgery before the sickness passed. It took two hours more for me to stop saying, "I won't have surgery tomorrow," and realize I *would* be having surgery tomorrow.

Charlie and Paul stayed at my side. I was calm now — deeply scared but quiet about it. Mitch Karlan and Ray Weston came in after dinner to find a patient who knew all about tomorrow and wanted more details about the surgery.

"I'm going to do a modified radical mastectomy," Mitch said.

That I was to have a radical mastectomy instead of a lumpectomy terrified me. I knew Mitch was a conservative surgeon; that he had decided to amputate meant I was in great danger. Mitch hadn't done a radical for a long time. He preferred whenever possible to perform a lumpectomy, where the tumor and all surrounding tissue are removed, leaving usually only a two-inch scar. Then a small incision is made in the armpit to remove the lymph nodes. I expected that was the worst I would have to face. But, God, my cancer had progressed to the point of a complete mastectomy.

Mitch was very solemn, an unusual expression on his habitually cheerful countenance. I didn't experience sharp, clean fear. It was more a blanket of smothering, clinging horror that couldn't be flung off, a new suit of clothes I could not remove.

"Okay," I said. "Do I have to stay in post-op and do I have to be sick? I want to get out of post-op as soon as possible, okay?"

They studied me a moment.

"The glass of water you drank in the morning was what made you sick. If you hadn't taken it, you wouldn't have been sick," Mitch said.

I clung to this. "Really? You mean I may not be sick tomorrow?"

"No, you don't have to be sick. Just have nothing by mouth tonight."

"I won't. I won't have anything if only I can get out of post-op quickly."

With a "Well, we'll see you tomorrow" (no "good luck" this time), they departed, leaving Charlie and me alone for the night.

The nurse wheeled in a cot for him; and after a while we

31

both lay down to try to sleep. I was given a sleeping pill and pain medication, but sleep was hard coming. I lay in bed terrified. I didn't want to die. Oh, my God, was there nothing I could do to escape my predicament? I wanted to cry but I couldn't. I was numb. Fear fitted over my emotions in a paralyzing grip. The night hours went by in orderly fashion as if nothing were wrong — but I was having a mastectomy tomorrow. Was that as it should be? I wanted to rip off the bandage covering the biopsy. I wanted to touch my breast while it was still with me; but, oh, God, there was an invader in there. I wanted to rip it out.

Oh, Charlie, wake up, come over here, I thought. But I said nothing.

Suddenly, too soon, morning came. The night nurse took my vital signs and went off duty. I looked over at Charlie. He was lying quietly. I broke the silence first, sitting up and looking over at my husband.

"You're awake," said Charlie.

"Yes. I've been awake, lying here waiting for you to wake up."

"I've been doing the same thing," he said.

I was overwhelmed. He looked so vulnerable. I had failed him by allowing myself to become this ill. He used to call me his golden girl. Would I still be?

I went over to his little cot and put my arms around him. "I love you."

"I love you, too," he said.

The day had begun.

My morning nurse came in. Sharon was blond, had an attractive, up personality, a perfect morning nurse. She did her best from the moment she entered the room to reassure a very anxious lady.

"Don't fight the anesthetic. Just let yourself go with it. Accept the woozy feeling." Sharon promised to come into the pre-op room until they took me into surgery. About three-thirty she said, "I have to give you a Demerol shot. They are coming for you now. It will help you relax."

I burst into tears. "No, please don't give me Demerol. Please don't give me Demerol. I'll relax," I sobbed.

My husband had his arms around me, unable to speak, while poor Sharon, the lovely, up nurse, just stuck the shot in my butt.

"I don't want to go, Charlie. Oh, I really don't want to go." I kept repeating that as I was wheeled into the corridor. A sympathetic face looked out from the bed in the next room. He knew I didn't want to go. He'd been and his head was shaved and bandaged. His eyes were compassionate.

We made it to the operating suite, where I was taken straight in. My anesthesiologist, Dr. Wender, was there. Ray was there. My husband was there. Sharon was there. My surgeon was on his way.

"Don't get me too woozy before Mitch gets here," I told Dr. Wender. I was holding Sharon's hand.

"Just relax," she said, "and go with it."

I really tried not to fight the anesthetic. Charlie stood beside me. Everyone wore a green cover over his head, mouth, clothes and shoes. By now I was suitably woozy. I was given more and more anesthetic surreptitiously through my IV. I knew by the telltale vapor of garlic in my throat. Mitch arrived and spoke cheerfully. I vaguely recall saying good-bye to Charlie and Sharon and being wheeled somewhere. Then I remember nothing until I was conscious of my chest being wrapped. I was regaining consciousness on the operating table. I was told later I had helped move myself onto a gurney.

I became fully conscious in the post-op room. I felt no pain and it was over. I didn't feel sick. They moved me quickly back to my room. No vomiting in the hall this time. What a relief! It was over. I'd made it. Compared with the day before, I had almost enjoyed it. Phew!

The nurse gave me a blue plastic toy with a suction piece and three balls in three upright plastic tubes.

"Suck air into your lungs, Jill, and hold the balls in the air as long as you can."

I looked at the gadget suspiciously. I tried tentatively. It had to hurt my chest, I thought. Somehow I took a big breath. Clack, clack, clack. I got all three balls in the air and held them there. This became my best trick. I played my game at hourly intervals to ensure my lungs were operating well after the anesthetic. I did it well. I was pleased with myself. The first hurdle was over. I had had my mastectomy. My arm was stiff and for a day or two it was a little swollen but, strangely enough, this time the pain was not that bad. There were drains in my chest with a pair of tubes leading to two blue drainage balls that rested at my side on a pillow.

"Don't pull them out, Jill," they cautioned me.

You bet I wouldn't.

Charlie arrived, bringing a home-cooked meal, and was rewarded by an exhibition of ball-clacking. He was as pleased and proud as if I'd just won a Grand Prix.

7

THE NEXT STEP. Now we were waiting for the pathology report. I was doing really well the day after surgery, walking, moving my arm and feeling hopeful. I knew some lymph nodes had been removed, but I didn't realize the significance of cancer in them until I talked to Mitch Karlan that day.

"Jill, if we find cancer in fewer than five nodes, we think it's not too bad a prognosis. But if five or more nodes have been affected, then it's bad. The statistics are not good," he said solemnly.

He was hopeful, however. During the operation he'd noticed an irregularity in only a single node. So, although I was scared, I was optimistic. We waited through the weekend and on Monday for the laboratory report. It finally came Tuesday evening. Charlie was with me in my hospital room. He answered the call from Mitch. I watched my husband's face. I wanted to know what he was being told. I inched up the bed closer to him and the telephone. I looked at Charlie. Did I see the same stricken look in his eyes that I'd seen only once before? There was a tense, nervous flutter in my stomach.

"You tell her, will you," Charlie said, handing me the phone.

"Well, Jill, they found it on eight nodes."

I gasped. "Eight! It's too many, it's too many. It's more than five!"

35

Fear and shock hit me. I hung up. Eight. That's too many. I cried and cried. God, was I going to die?

Within minutes, Ray Weston came rushing into the room. I learned later he had known the results all day and waited outside my room for an hour before Mitch called. Mitch thought it was his place to tell me himself.

"It's too many, Ray," I cried. "I expected one, or at the most three, but eight is too many." Again, I was inconsolable. Eight cancerous nodes meant *chemotherapy*.

"I don't want to die. I can't leave Zuleika. She's only twelve. I don't want to leave Zuleika, and I don't want to leave Charlie. Ray, promise me you won't let me die in pain. Please promise you won't let me die in pain."

I was trapped. "I want to get out of here." I searched the room frantically. I met two pairs of scared eyes — Charlie's and Ray's. They thought I was going to get up and try it.

"I don't want to tell my nurses. I don't want them to know."

At that, I saw Sharon hurry from the room. In the few days the nurses and I had been together we had become close. They, too, were waiting for the pathology report. I couldn't face telling them the truth. Gradually, my sobbing quieted, and Ray was able to talk to me.

"You are going to get well," he told me. "You must believe that. You are going to have six months of chemotherapy, and you are going to recover. The doctor of oncology is coming to see you. He will explain chemotherapy. Don't be put off by his appearance; he dresses funny, sort of like Charlie."

At that moment, into the room came a slight man in corduroy trousers, a shirt, tie and jacket. He carried a man's shoulder bag. His hair was a little long and curly. His face was sensitive. He studied me with understanding eyes, eyes that told me he had come to help, eyes that told me he was familiar with this moment. His job was treating cancer patients, which I now was. He sat beside me on the bed.

"My name is Michael Van Scoy Mosher. I'm the oncologist."

Charlie said, "Jesus, we don't have to call you that, do we?"

The doctor said, "You can call me Michael if you like." He looked me straight in the eyes.

"It's too many," I said. "It's on eight nodes."

I became immediately demanding. My brain was racing. Words came out quickly. "I need help. Tell me about chemotherapy. Will my hair fall out? Will I be sick?"

He told me, "Everybody is different." Maybe my hair would not fall out, but I should have a wig standing by. He told me they would wrap my head in ice to close off the hair follicles during treatment. This might help. They would give me medication for nausea. Some people didn't get sick.

I stared at him, sensing his quiet strength and understanding.

"How do you give it to me?"

"In an IV injection."

"Not a drip?"

"No."

"How long does it take?"

"About three or four minutes."

"I'm very scared of it."

"I know you are. Everybody is. You'll find the first treatment is the most frightening. It's fear of the unknown. But you need it. You will have one treatment every three weeks for six months."

Charlie was shocked. "Can she take these treatments in Vermont?"

I knew what he was thinking. We had spent the last eleven summers at our country home, Zuleika Farm East. Charlie *needs* the isolation of Vermont, almost to survive. With one step he finds himself alone in an environment that provides instant solitude, freedom from the noise, the distractions and superficiality of the city.

"I can't go to Vermont," I cried. "I can't! I won't! I must stay here. I need my doctors."

37

Michael never took his eyes from me. He discussed the need to have bone marrow and liver scans. I didn't want to take them. I was frightened I would have an adverse reaction to the dye they inject and, more important, I was afraid I might be given more devastating news. Cancer could be in my bones. I had been so disappointed by the recent pathology report that I knew it was important for me to regroup and rebuild my inner resources before I faced anything else. I asked Michael if the treatment would be any different if the cancer had spread to my bones.

"The same," he said.

"So I have nothing to gain at the moment by taking the scans, only disappointment."

Michael said, "Okay, I can go with that. You will have to take them later. We'll need them as a baseline, but for now we'll leave it."

I had made my first decision about my health and my own life since entering the hospital. And as much as it was possible at the moment, I felt good. Suddenly, I knew I would rebuild, but I needed time. I had been bombarded with bad news for days. I was sorting and assimilating those blows. I was going to handle it. It was going to take a lot of energy and personal will. God, God, God. It was true. Faced with a life-threatening situation, you *did* call for God.

I found an ally in Michael. During that first visit, he introduced me to the idea of holistic healing. I desperately needed some guidance, an organized pattern by which to start waging war on cancer.

Michael explained that holistic healing was a means of treating the patient as a whole entity and not just dealing with the sick or injured part. In other words, it approaches the patient not only physiologically by also psychologically.

I looked at this man who had come to help me and said, "I could never do that thing where you imagine your white blood cells gobbling up the cancer cells. I don't have the powers of concentration."

As I finished the sentence, I realized that that was the first thing he was about to suggest.

I stared into his eyes. He nodded.

"I could do it!" I said. I changed my mind that fast. I knew I needed all the help I could get.

After Michael left, my husband went home to dinner with Zuleika and Katrina, leaving Paul with me. We were quiet and sad. We spoke softly for forty-five minutes, when into the room, unannounced, came a red-haired doctor in hospital whites. He had accompanied Dr. Karlan on a couple of visits, so I trusted his intentions.

He said, "Good evening. Have you heard your pathology report yet?"

Still full of support and understanding from Ray and Michael, I was trusting and vulnerable. "Yes, they told me it was on eight lymph nodes. Of course, I'm very upset. I decided not to have the liver and bone scans."

"May I ask why?" he asked chidingly.

"Well, my doctor said the treatment would be the same anyway, and I'm too disappointed right now to face the possibility of another disappointment."

"Well," he said, "as long as you have them sooner or later."

"Why? What difference does it make? The treatment is the same if it has gone into the bones. I am frightened that may be the case. Why would I want to have the scans?"

His answer hit Paul and me like a cannonball. "Well, you may want to change your life plans."

Whap! Life plans!

Paul said, "Wait a minute. Are you saying if it's in her bones it's terminal?"

"Yes," he said. "But you're feeling fine now, for the time being, so do what you want. Try to enjoy yourself, okay?"

With that, he turned and left the room. My son rushed after him. Paul grabbed him by the shoulders in the hallway and spun him around.

"How long will she have if it's in her bones?"

"I can't say."

"Well, give me a ballpark figure."

He didn't want to reply. Paul was desperate. "I'm asking you. Give me a ballpark figure."

"Well, all right," the doctor said. "Maybe five years."

Paul returned to the room.

"You went after that doctor, didn't you?"

"No, I just went outside for a moment."

I looked at my son. "Come on, Paul. What did he say?"

"Well, he said a ballpark figure on your life expectancy, if it's in your bones, is five years."

God! I was giddy from the horror of the whole evening. I was now sure it was in my bones. Paul and I sat together in quiet acceptance of my plight. After a while Paul prepared to leave to teach his scuba-diving class. "Paul, I know you're upset, but don't bend the whole class, okay?"

He left with a wan smile and I settled down with my night nurse and my thoughts. If I had five years, I could see my daughter into her eighteenth year. She was twelve right now but in August she would be a teenager. Could I count the five years, including her birthday? I must be around as Zuleika went through the difficult teens. I must. I pursued those morbid thoughts the rest of the night.

8

I WAS CHANGED. I had cancer. Everyone reacted to it and me differently.

Oh my God, those sympathetic eyes. Those fearful, sympathetic eyes. Goose bumps would prickle up on my arms every time I locked eyes with a doctor or nurse I hoped would be my savior. I found without excption, as far as the doctors and medical workers were concerned, their attitude toward me as a cancer patient was one of compassion with a touch of "God, I'm glad it's not me." I knew they were hoping I would produce a "good attitude," the panacea for cancer recovery. Unlike the bromide Physician, heal thyself, I could have sworn they were saying, Patient, heal thyself. It was all there to read in their eyes. Now, like Dorothy in the *Wizard of Oz,* all I had to do was click my ruby slippers three times, say, "There's no place like home," and find myself a "good attitude."

I found myself role-playing. I saw the ugly possibility of the power I could wield through the careful use of subtle implication. I haven't long to live, so you should do what I want. I have cancer, remember? I knew that it would be a powerful weapon. I also saw it was one that could make loved ones almost hate me. At the same time, they would feel guilty, trapped by me, the cancer victim. As much as possible, I told myself, no role-playing, no manipulation. I wanted my relationships to be honest and free.

Charlie, his presence filling the hospital room with quiet

stoicism, brought me yellow roses. He told me later that his deepest thought was how to help me adjust to losing my breast and how, above all, to appear to be optimistic. It was almost impossible for him to accept that this situation was beyond his control.

My twenty-one-year-old son, Jason, found it hard to visit. He stood outside the room, literally bouncing off the walls, winding up, getting ready to come in. Once inside, he was falsely up, cheerful and full of jokes. He caromed around in a jerky, spastic way. A typical Jason greeting: "Hey, Mama, what's happening?"

I'd reply, "Hi, Jayce, how are you?"

I longed to put my arms around him and say it was okay, I wasn't going to die. But he was too slippery. He'd never allow himself to be caught alone with me, and he never let up on his hyper, stand-up comic act. After a quick kiss, he stayed on the other side of the room, moving around, joking with the nurses, doing anything not to acknowledge what was going on. We are very close, and it broke my heart to watch him. I knew he was totally unable to cope. My poor Jason. Later, many months down the road, he was to confront those feelings, but only when I was better. Only then could he hold me, crying.

"I was so scared, Mom. I thought I was going to lose you."

Valentine found it hard to visit in the beginning, but he coped better than Jason. Val sat by the bed, unable at first to do anything but stare at me or at the floor. But it was easier to reach him; there was no act to cut through, just the look of abject misery. I could hold Val, at least for as long as he could bend his six-foot-seven frame over the bed. He came to feel so at home during visits he would eat and visit at the same time. Colleen, my afternoon nurse, would ask when Val was coming so he could clean out the tiny refrigerator for her. He was always famished. Val is slender, so the food seemed to disappear into a vacuum. He would eat my leftover lunch, half a tuna sandwich, any fruit, half-finished yogurt, candy — anything.

Zuleika visited with Charlie, wearing her gray school uniform, her hair in a ponytail, navy blue socks sliding down into her scuffed brown penny loafers. She was quiet.

She said, "Hi, Mom," and bent stiffly to kiss me.

How I wanted to pick her up, put her in bed with me, hold her warm body next to mine as I had when she was a very little girl. Instead, I stroked her soft cheek and smiled at her, saying, "Hello, Baba. How was your day?"

I saw that with a quick glance she took in the blue trailing tubes I was trying to conceal under the sheets, the top of my bandage and the little doll that she had given me a year earlier lying on the pillow beside my head.

She seemed to believe me when I said I was going to be all right. Why not? I'd never lied to her. She was cramming for her end-of-term finals. Charlie helped Zuleika with her studies in the room, grilling her over and over again. One day Val, having eaten everything in sight, became bored with Charlie's drill. He did everything to distract Zuleika by playing with a large, life-sized stuffed monkey puppet that Paul had given me. Val sat behind Charlie, out of his line of sight, and made the monkey look curiously around the room; its eyes seemed alive as they peered in the direction Val aimed the head. The monkey (I'd named him Bernie) had a cocky, almost wicked expression. Val pointed the puppet in Charlie's direction as he relentlessly grilled Zuleika. She tried hard not to see Bernie, but finally weakened and snuck a look. Charlie saw her concentration dissolve and followed Zuleika's stare. As he did, Bernie produced a huge, long, rumbling belch. Val, a master of burps, had stored air for just the right moment. As Charlie turned in irritation, Val let it rip. Burrrppp! Insolent Bernie! We all broke up; laughter filled the hospital room. Paul and Charlie laughed until tears rolled down their cheeks. Val, irrepressible Valentine. When he was a boy, about to be reprimanded by Charlie's stern "Val!" he would chirp optimistically, "I know you love me, right?" Charlie could never get angry with Val, a most-welcome visitor. He made me laugh.

Charlie's twenty-nine-year-old daughter, Suzanne, visited

and came straight to the point. "I'm frightened. You've got cancer. Are you going to die? I love you and I'm so scared."

I looked into her slanted, golden eyes — so like her father's — and said, "No, I'm not; not yet anyway, so stop worrying."

Katrina came, and Tony, Charlie's handsome twenty-three-year-old son, bringing little gifts and anxious, dark eyes. Still I was able to hold all of them, to reach them. It was only Jason who was in deep trouble. He wouldn't, couldn't talk about it. Not with me, not with any of the family. The rest of us had no choice but to let Jason fight his devils his own way, but it hurt to watch him.

Charlie's sister Catherine called to say her entire church was praying for me. The energy of all those people praying had to be very powerful. Charlie's brother Dempsey and his wife, Anne, visited and sent loving cards, adding their prayers.

My brother, John, spoke to me every night from his home in Canada, usually bringing a touch of his own off-the-wall humor. One night a couple of days after surgery, he asked why my surgeon didn't rearrange my good left breast in the middle of my chest. Then I could wear it hanging out of my V-necked dresses, starting a new fashion.

One morning I read an article Michael Van Scoy Mosher, my oncologist, had written about chemotherapy and its side effects. It seemed I would be sick the day of the treatment. My hair would probably fall out. The prospect seemed remote. Not like it was really happening to me. I couldn't imagine myself bald. However, a part of me could, because I called my hairdresser and asked him to make a wig. It was strange how selective my thoughts were. I could believe I might die, but I couldn't believe my hair would fall out.

A few days after the operation, Mitch Karlan changed my dressing. I was scared of this moment, and squeamish. I didn't want to see myself. I told Charlie to stand in the corner and look out the window. I had my hands in the air as the dressing was cut down the back and removed. Oh, what a strange, empty feeling I had on my right side.

"It looks good, Jill. The skin is beautiful." Mitch covered an area under my arm where the drain was inserted. "Now you can look."

I peered down with my eyes only, then with my head. It wasn't too bad. There was a patch of tape over the incision. Where my breast had been was a flat surface with a scar running just below my armpit across what would have been the middle of my breast. The area above the scar was smooth and tanned. I had no scar in the middle of my chest. I saw I could wear low, V-necked dresses.

Dr. Karlan allowed me to inspect myself for a few seconds. Then he told Charlie to come over. He did. Charlie said it didn't look too bad to him. Somehow, Mitch had covered part of my chest with a gauze pad, so Charlie didn't see it all. We sent Charlie back to his corner while I was rebandaged.

When this was done, I told Mitch about my experience with the red-haired doctor. He let out a snort of laughter. "He's only an intern. God, when will these interns learn?" Mitch proceeded to tell about an intern who gave a woman a pelvic examination the night before her surgery and declared he could feel nothing wrong. The woman's surgeon came to the hospital at midnight to reassess her X rays and assure her the operation was necessary. It turned out the intern had never given a pelvic before.

"Well," I said, "I guess I'm lucky I didn't get a pelvic. I feel a little better." But it didn't relieve my fear of bone scans. Mitch said, "It's not in your bones. Stop worrying. We just need the scans for the future, as a baseline." He left the room, probably to find the lamentable intern.

I had learned a lesson. Don't listen to people just because they work in hospitals — doctors, nurses, whomever. Protect yourself from misinformation and gratuitous advice. Learn to say, "When I want your opinion, I'll ask for it." Learn to say, "I don't want to talk about it." Learn to say, "I don't want to hear about your uncle Henry, your aunt Lillian, or your friend's mother." I was becoming stronger.

Two drains remained in the incision pumping out fluid.

45

One was under my armpit and another close to the center of my chest, over my sternum. The drains were operated by a small electric pump that often failed. My nurses were forever tinkering with it, squeezing the little balls that collected the fluid. The squeezing created suction, a strange, gurgly feeling; not painful, but unpleasant. The blue balls, draining red and yellow fluid, stayed with me for days. I put them in the pocket of my robe to walk around the corridors, each day venturing farther. I took hip baths with the balls tucked into the top of my bandage. You can get accustomed to almost anything. I was certainly used to my balls. God, it was like a bad sex change operation — two balls in my pocket and one breast gone.

I loved mornings in the hospital and always felt up. I tired in the afternoons and usually took a five-minute nap. It was curious how five minutes seemed to revive me. I hated nights. It was hard to sleep lying on my back, propped up, with my right arm lying on a pillow. I was scared and it was at night I thought my most grisly thoughts. I couldn't read or distract myself with television. I could only hang on until morning. I had now been in the hospital seven days. The hospital's rough open-backed nightshirt had been replaced by a pretty nightgown and matching robe of my own. Contrary to what I had expected, I was feeling little pain and moving quite easily around the room. Each morning I arose with new hope. I exercised my arm. Ouch! It was still stiff and painful. I had developed phlebitis from a needle that had drawn blood from my right arm the day after surgery, before I had been instructed, "Don't let anybody take anything from this arm." So I was sore. However, I exercised, walked, bathed and organized my bedside table and, most important, saw Michael, the oncologist, daily.

He stopped by one morning and said, "Remember, after chemotherapy your hair will grow back and most women say it returns thicker."

"Does it always fall out?"

"Well, in a few cases it doesn't. But I would buy a wig just in case," he said again.

Michael scribbled on my chart, and then we discussed holistic healing again. Although it was a new concept to me, I dearly wanted to start as soon as possible. Ray Weston's wife, Lynne, had worked with holistic therapy during her long battle with cancer, so Ray encouraged me in my pursuit of further knowledge of the subject. I wanted to see a psychologist or a psychiatrist for therapy, too. Michael told me he would give me the names of some people. I wanted detailed instructions on how to apply my mind to healing myself. Michael gave me the name of Dr. O. Carl Simonton. Ray had also told me about him. He was an oncologist who fostered the self-help technique in overcoming cancer. I decided to get Dr. Simonton's book, *Getting Well Again*, co-authored by Stephanie Matthews-Simonton and James Creighton.

At the same time, I became superstitious. I always knocked on wood. I carried a wooden pencil over my ear and knocked on it a dozen times a day. I made everyone else knock on wood, too. When I misplaced the pencil I would panic until it was recovered. What I needed was a wooden bracelet, one made of good, strong wood that I could wear all the time.

Charlie visited every day, quietly watchful, bringing news from home. He finally told Zuleika that we wouldn't be going to Vermont this summer. She had been very disappointed. But Charlie told her, "Mom needs us now. She's always been there for us. Now it's our turn to be there for her."

And, finally, just eight days after my mastectomy, I went home to start my new life with cancer and one breast.

9

MY LIFE IN THE HOSPITAL had been narrowed down to one small, secure environment, everything within reach — like being in a cocoon. Now faced with my home again, it seemed altogether too large and spread out. I didn't know where to settle. I was frightened, intimidated about being cut loose. For a moment I wondered if I had come home too soon.

Charlie, full of bounding energy, walked beside me while I slowly and painfully crept up the long flight of stairs to the front door.

Then he asked, "Where do you want to sit?"

He was carrying a large bag. Charlie had packed for me and had overlooked nothing — my books, greeting cards, vomit dish and, yes, he had even packed my blue clack-clack balls. I was glad I had sent my goldfish and balloons, which friends had brought, down to the children's ward.

I stood in the foyer. The sitting room looked much too far away. I could hear Zuleika and some young friends splashing around in the swimming pool. But I didn't want to sit outside.

"I think I'll go up to my dressing room."

Charlie sprang up the stairs with my things. I immediately regretted my decision. The banister rail was on my right. So was my surgery.

"I changed my mind, Charlie," I called weakly. "I think I will go into the sitting room after all."

In a moment he was back at my side, helping me along the corridor to the sitting room, where he deposited me on a couch. All the family came in to see me, delighted I was home.

My brother, John, had flown from Canada for my first weekend at home. He and Charlie happily engaged themselves at the pool table while the rest of us enjoyed tea and cookies, talking and joking as if we were celebrating a family birthday or graduation.

I looked good. I'd lost weight. It was flattering, and my eyes seemed larger. I thought of the shadows underneath them as romantic. I might have lost a breast, but my legs were fantastic. By now, I was definitely feeling okay. It was the honeymoon period with the disease.

I enjoyed watching Charlie and John shoot pool. Charlie seemed contented, lost in the game. John kept the jokes coming, removing his shoes and sliding around the tiled floor in his socks, making perfect shots as he skidded from position to position around the billiard table. He looked up and said, "Jill, you have a visitor. It's either a concert violinist or a doctor."

In the doorway stood Ray Weston. Yes, he did look like a violinist — tall, bearded, artistic, carrying a black bag.

"Hi, Ray."

He kissed me. "Hi, dear. How are you? I talked to your nurse. She told me you had a good night."

"Yes, I feel fine, Ray. If it's all right, I'd like to have a glass of wine with dinner tonight."

Ray studied me carefully. Charlie looked up from his shot. "Will that mix with the pain and sleep medication she's taking?"

Ray considered, then told me, "All right, dear, you can have a little wine."

"Yippee! A party."

49

Ray stayed long enough to have a cup of tea and to watch the end of the pool match. Then he kissed me good-bye and said he would see me tomorrow.

I left to go to my dressing room to change. I still wore a large dressing and wraparound bandage that circled my upper right arm, my neck and down across the empty right chest. It was hard to dress. But with a soft, baggy, silk man-style shirt and a very loose jacket, I managed. I dressed awkwardly and slowly. There was considerable pain when I used my right shoulder and arm, making the act of putting on a shirt challenging and totally exhausting. I suddenly panicked, overwhelmed with the reality of my situation. I breathed in shallow, rapid gulps. My heart pounded, thrashing in my chest. I looked at myself in the mirror. A terrified, haunted face glared back at me. I flew out of the room and into Charlie's large walk-in closet, where he was dressing for dinner. I began incoherently throwing words at him, words of misery and fear.

He was hungry, overstressed. He felt under attack. Was I going to take it out on him every time I panicked? Because I had cancer? He shook his fists in the air in frustration. He believed I was angry with him because I had cancer and he didn't. The energy in the closet was dangerously close to blowing the whole roof off. I had pushed Charlie too far.

Somehow, I controlled myself; I begged him to forgive me, begged him to understand. "Please, Charlie, I'm just so scared. Please, Charlie," I sobbed.

"Okay, leave me alone now. I have to dress. We're late for our dinner reservation. Your timing is all wrong; everyone is waiting for us. Go finish getting ready."

Good food and a few drinks calmed us both. I sat glued to Charlie's side in the booth at the restaurant. I was weak, drained emotionally and physically. I was very needy, very scared. But, my God, Charlie was even more scared, more needy. Charlie, red-eyed and wiped out, returned my gaze tenderly, his eyes penetrating deep into mine. I felt his love. Charlie didn't respond to my need in a textbook perfect way, but how could I expect him to? He was in big trouble. His whole life was disrupted, his being violated by an unexpected, noncompromising disease. "Oh, Charlie, I love you so much," I whispered in his ear.

Our bond was deep; I knew we would make it. But I realized I needed outside help. I wanted the man I loved to be the one who saved me, helped me, picked me up, babied me, listened to the outpouring of rage and grief. But he just couldn't, at least not in the way I needed. I never doubted Charlie loved me, but it seemed too difficult for him to accept the fact that my life was in jeopardy. After all, I was younger. I believed he had always thought he would die first. He was reeling from shock. He needed time to recover. We both were in psychological pain.

Even as I hurt, I felt his sustaining love. Over the years Charlie and I had been through so much together, the pain of breaking up two households, melding two families, traveling, working — those years had created a bond. I knew he would stay by my side and see me through it in his own way. It would be "till death us do part."

I felt the fight rising in me. I knew it would be a long battle. I didn't know how, but I was going to win it. I was not going down easy. Damn you, cancer. I was going to get it all back — my health, strength, looks — everything.

Two weeks after my surgery, one long night, I had trouble sleeping. Charlie woke up, aware I was restless, and he stretched his arm toward me.

"Having trouble, baby? Come here, put your head on my shoulder."

I did. I always said it was the best place in the world. I loved lying with my head on Charlie's shoulder. Then, sliding down to his chest, I would listen to the sound of his heartbeat and synchronize my breathing with his. This night I felt especially close to him. It was so soon after my surgery, and I was still quite sore. Lying on my right side, where the breast had been removed, was still uncomfortable, but the discomfort did not diminish my deep pleasure. Lying there made me aware I still felt like *me*. The closeness, the physical proximity, brought a sexual response.

Charlie said, "You'll have to move. You're too close to me."

Nothing could prevent me from staying right where I was. Then, in the middle of a night I had thought was too long, our love life continued. I never really thought it wouldn't; perhaps I should have. I should not have taken Charlie for granted.

I had heard so many stories about husbands being turned off by their wives' surgeries and wives disgusted with themselves and the sight of the mastectomy scar. I had read Betty Rollin's book *First, You Cry,* but I went through none of the self-conscious discomfort she described. She wrote, "If you feel deformed, it's hard to feel sexy. For me, anyway, feeling sexy had a lot to do with feeling beautiful. . . ."

I realized how lucky I was that Charlie and I could pick up and resume a normal, healthy sex life so soon after my surgery. That was not to be one of my problems.

I dreaded my first chemotherapy session, scheduled three weeks after surgery. The date was still two weeks distant but it occupied my thoughts. I was truly scared of anything given intravenously. I knew once a chemical was in my system no one could get it out. The poison that killed cancer cells also damaged healthy cells. Maybe I would have an allergic reaction and die during the treatment. Nothing anyone said made it less oppressive.

It was strange, too, not being in Vermont in June. Charlie was sad and lost. He missed New England. We rented a small house on the beach in Malibu where we could relax and put some sort of order back into our lives. It was a cozy house with a roomy veranda overlooking the blue Pacific and a spacious sitting room with two comfortable couches facing a large window with a vista of the sea. The master bedroom was big and airy. It had once been occupied by Julie Andrews and her director husband, Blake Edwards. Nine months earlier

Blake had seen me in a restaurant with my broken leg in its metal brace.

"Let me put my hands on the leg," he'd said. "Sometimes I've been able to help. I have power in my hands to heal."

So saying, he placed his hands on my leg; I felt the warmth flow through. I stood awkwardly in the middle of the crowded dining room, somewhat embarrassed but willing to try anything. I had feared my leg would never heal. After a time Blake removed his hands and wished me well. It could have been due to Blake or the electromagnetic impulse machine, but the leg healed a month later.

I told Charlie, "Maybe it is a good sign that Blake once occupied this room." I liked the house. It felt right. We rented it for four months.

On the way home, after agreeing to take the house for the summer, we stopped and I bought a large wooden bracelet and had my hair washed. I told the girl at the beauty parlor I had hurt my shoulder, keeping my surgery secret to prevent newspapers from printing the story. I was happy for the first time in weeks. I had found a house, bought my wooden bracelet and had my hair washed. It had been a good day, full of small triumphs.

When I returned to Bel Air, Paul was waiting with bad news.

"Mom, reporters have been calling all day. The *National Enquirer* mostly. They know you've been in the hospital. I tried to fend them off. I said if you'd been seen there, it was because I'd been ill, that you were just visiting me. But it's only a matter of time before they print a story. You'd better call Grandma and Grandpa."

It distressed me to think of my elderly parents so far away. My father had suffered a stroke, which left him unable to speak. He could say only, "Lo, lo, lo." His right arm and leg were paralyzed but this didn't prevent him from exercising and gardening. My mother, a gallant soul, coped wonderfully. She and my father were proud of me and John. They believed everything was right with the world if we were well and happy. Now this. I couldn't call her. I telephoned John and asked him to break the news before the press called Mummy. I didn't want her reading about my illness in the papers. John called just in time. He beat the first inquiry from a reporter by two hours. My mother telephoned immediately, full of encouragement, recommending a film she'd seen called *Champion,* about a steeplechase jockey, Bob Champion, and his fight against cancer. He had not only recovered, he had gone on to win the Grand National, the most grueling steeplechase in the world.

My little mother was an inspiration. "You're tough, Jill; you come from strong stock. You stick it out. Take the chemotherapy no matter how much you hate it. It will be worth it in the end."

I promised her I would. I was so anxious to minimize her anxiety that, listening, Charlie told me later I sounded as if I were advocating breast amputation as quite the thing to do, a new, fun experience. Mummy told me she loved me. Then she put my father on.

"Lo, lo," a weak, choked-up voice said.

I nearly broke down. "I'm fine, Daddy, really. I'm fine. Thousands of women have this operation, Daddy. It's nothing. I didn't have any pain. I'm fine — I really am." Oh, God, now he was crying. "I love you, Daddy, take care of yourself. Please don't cry. I'm going to be fine."

So now they knew; now everybody knew. Maybe it was for the best. I wouldn't have to pretend. The story was printed in the *National Enquirer:* Jill Bronson has only one tit. I would have to live with that. A small inner voice said, "As long as you live, you silly fool, as long as you live."

10

IT WAS NEARLY THREE WEEKS after my surgery. I went to Michael's office to make an appointment for my first chemotherapy.

Michael gave me prescriptions for Compazine suppositories, to suppress nausea, and Decadron, anti-inflammatory tablets. I insisted he take me to the room where he would give me the treatment. I made him show me the hypodermic needle and the syringe that would be used when I received the chemicals. I asked what he would do if I had an allergic reaction.

Michael said, "I would give you Adrenalin. But, Jill, the chemicals are not the sort of drugs people react to allergically."

I was not reassured. I had been the one-in-a-million exception too often in the past. I asked him everything I could think of. I took the little white card with my appointment and prescriptions written on it: *take one Decadron every six hours starting the morning of the treatment. After treatment, one Compazine suppository every four hours.* A desperate calm and terrible resignation took over. The treatment was scheduled for the following Thursday. God, it was really happening.

Determined to use all the holistic healing techniques I could, I began listening to taped lectures by Dr. O. Carl Simonton, the oncologist whose studies demonstrated how much more progress was made by cancer patients who used visualization techniques while meditating. Dr. Simonton advised meditating three times a day — once in the morning upon arising, once after lunch, and then again before bedtime. The meditation consisted of going into a deep state of relaxation, then imagining cancer in a way that made sense, perhaps as a series of black spots or a lump of raw liver. The next step was to imagine the white blood cells as perhaps a ferocious dog or a school of fish with large teeth, which set about viciously destroying the cancer.

Thursday came. I awoke bilious and with a bad headache. I dressed myself and carefully made up my face as if I had a social engagement of some importance.

"Hang in there, kid," Michael said when he saw me. "Let's just get this started, okay?"

He left me and Charlie alone in the treatment room. I had never been more frightened of anything in my life. The fear was all-consuming, paralyzing. The nurse placed a rubber tourniquet around my head. Over that she put a heavy ice helmet, to help prevent loss of hair. I sat rigidly in a wooden chair while my head was chilled. Then Michael entered carrying three large bottles. I looked away but not before I glimpsed one container of dark green fluid and another of red. Fluorouracil and Adriamycin, I had been told. The third liquid was Cytoxan.

Michael helped me lie on the table. My head wobbled on my shoulders from the weight of the ice helmet. I looked into my husband's eyes and held his hand. My feet twitched convulsively.

I said to Charlie, "Talk to me about Zuleika." He tried hard. Michael slid the needle into my vein with the dexterity of a skilled swordsman. Looking like a turn-of-the-century poet, with his long, curly hair, he injected the drugs into my body while Charlie desperately tried to talk about Zuleika and anything else he could think of. It seemed to take hours.

One vial was gone. Michael began the second.

"This may make you feel a slight flush in your face, Jill."

"Oh, no, I'll hate that." However, no flush. Michael was

nearly finished. I felt him moving something around and panicked. "What are you doing now?"

"Putting on a Band-Aid. It's over."

"It's over? Really?"

It had taken less than ten minutes.

"Yes. Just lie there for a while and you can go home."

"Oh, please let me sit up," I said. "I feel so helpless lying down."

He helped me sit up, and the nurse removed the ice helmet and tourniquet. What a relief. It was over. I could smile. Oh, God, it was over. I said good-bye and went home.

I floated on air in the car. It was done. I survived. One down and only seven more chemos to go. I was suffused by feelings of reprieve and relief. "Oh, Charlie, I was so scared. I was sure I would have an allergic reaction to the drugs and go into a coma. I was so scared it would kill me." Michael had told me everyone was scared. I was by no means the most frightened person he had treated. At least my veins hadn't retracted. I thought my veins would have done just that if they had known they could.

We pulled into our Bel Air driveway. Home again. The house looked familiar, steady, unshakable. It seemed to be sending me the message — "You're home again, Jill, everything is going to be okay." I walked unsteadily up the stairs to the entryway, then into the downstairs powder room. I paused briefly at the ornate, gold-framed mirror to look at myself. Everything seemed to be all right. I looked the same. I sat down on the toilet and put my head in my hands from sheer nervous exhaustion. I'd had my first chemotherapy. Yea me. I'd survived. I peed with relief, then I stood up and pressed the button to flush the toilet. I looked down. My heart paused in its steady rhythm and gave a startled thump. The water in the bowl was bright red, a sickening, oily-looking red. The drugs had gone right through me. I had read in some chemotherapy literature that red urine could occur, but I had forgotten about it. Now I had what my mother would have called a rude awakening. My body didn't seem to be my own. Unfamiliar things were going on at all levels. Still, the first chemo was over. I'd make it.

I experienced such relief at that that I was actually happy. I ate a light dinner with my family and called my brother to tell him so far, so good.

I took my pills and religiously used the suppositories. Wiped out from tension and apprehension, I went to bed early. I was still taking Percocet pain medication and a sleeping pill, so I slept until six. I awoke feeling — whoops — sick. I slipped quietly out of bed and went downstairs to wait it out. I vomited twice; the rest of the time I just felt miserable and exhausted. As the day wore on I felt a bit better, but still fragile. I spoke to Ray Weston and Michael. I wanted to see Zuleika ride in a horse show that evening. The arena was a forty-five-minute drive from home. Michael said, "Yes, I don't see any reason why you shouldn't go." By four that afternoon I had pulled myself together. Still feeling fragile, I set off with Charlie for the show.

En route, I began to think this was not a good idea. As we negotiated a winding road I became woozy.

"You don't look too good," Charlie said. "I think we should turn back."

I wasn't sure. I wasn't sure of much at all, actually. I was sort of out of it. And, yup, sick.

"Maybe you'd better turn around," I said.

No sooner spoken, and Charlie had turned back down the winding glen, than I began to grow numb. What was happening in my throat? My tongue was numb. I had trouble swallowing. My tongue began to protrude. We were near home but I felt so ill I wondered if I would make it. By the time we pulled into our driveway I could hardly speak, but I managed, "Charlie, get Ray Weston — it's an emergency."

My arm was numb now. I walked up two flights of stairs to our front door, then two more to our bedroom. Charlie called Ray, who said he was on his way.

I trembled all over, sure I was dying. Hurry up, Ray. I tried to relax. I tried to stay calm. Charlie called Mitchell Karlan, who was out of town. We contacted his associate, Dr. Robert Uyeda, who also rushed over.

Charlie then called Michael, who listened to the symptoms and said, "It sounds like a Compazine reaction. Do you have any Benadryl in the house?"

We didn't. My legs were trembling violently. I didn't know how much longer I could handle this dreadful attack. I thought I would choke, my tongue was so thick and numb.

While Charlie spoke to Michael, Ray walked in. Dr. Uyeda arrived. He and Ray examined me.

"Calm down," Ray said. "You're going to be all right."

With my tongue paralyzed and protruding, I was almost unable to speak, but I croaked, "Help me. Do something to make it stop, Ray."

He needed Benadryl. He called two pharmacies. Neither delivered. It was late on a Friday night. I couldn't believe it. I was dying and no one delivered. Charlie drove to a drugstore for the Benadryl. Oh, Charlie, hurry up, I thought.

Ray looked at me sitting on the bed in my shorts and man's shirt with my tongue sticking out. He smiled affectionately and said to Dr. Uyeda, as if I weren't there, "Isn't she cute? She looks like a little pixie, doesn't she? Just like a kid."

I was desperate, wondering how much longer I could hold on. I couldn't speak. My tongue and throat were paralyzed. I stared at Ray in terror. I wanted to say, "*Please,* do something. I need help, not compliments." I felt as if I were going to pass out. Only my will kept me from going under.

Charlie returned more quickly than I thought possible. Ray injected me with Benadryl, and I took two pills and lay down, waiting to feel better.

It took hours for the Benadryl to work. Eventually, I did stop shaking and my tongue retracted into my mouth. But the nervy, spastic jumping of my knees and hips went on until late into the night.

The next day I was almost back to normal. I was tired but all the symptoms had disappeared. I had had my first chemotherapy. Next time I would definitely take *nothing* for nausea — certainly not Compazine.

11

MICHAEL ARRANGED FOR ME to have a private meeting with Dr. O. Carl Simonton, the oncologist and holistic practitioner. Here was the wizard I had been looking for. It was with hope in my heart, wearing my version of ruby slippers — red tennis shoes — that I carefully hauled myself up into the cab of Paul's truck. My dog Cassie hopped into the flatbed behind us, wagging her tail happily at the prospect of an outing. We drove up Mulholland Drive to the flower-banked garden of the house where Simonton was staying, parked and walked to the house, leaving Cassie in the truck.

We were shown into a small, comfortable den. Within minutes Dr. Simonton appeared. With gray hair and a gray beard, he was a tall, robust, teddy bear of a man wearing gray slacks and a blue sweater, which matched his open, kind blue eyes. Breezing into the room with an air of confidence, he shook my hand and Paul's. He filled me with hope, and I had an urge to jump into his lap, saying, "Save me! Save me!"

Instead, I said, "I read your book and I think it's only fair to tell you that I look on you as sort of a savior."

Dr. Simonton rubbed his beard and chuckled. "Well, thank you," he said.

He had a large order to fill. Pulling his leather chair close to where I was sitting on a couch, he began talking to me in a quiet, measured way. He questioned me carefully about my life, my family and my career. I found myself telling him how busy I'd been, about Katrina's mother's death, my brother, John's, brain tumor, how responsible I felt for my parents and how my father's illness worried me. I also told him about my ordeal with consecutive leg injuries, and how for a long time before my illness I had been driving myself, giving priority to duties and other people's problems, putting off the things I really wanted to do, simply not putting aside enough time for the quiet and solitude that I craved. I felt I was indispensable to my house, family, friends and animals. I was convinced I was the only one that could do all the immeasurable things with which I filled my day. I had been using caffeine when I was tired so that I could keep going, painkillers such as Ascriptin A/D so that I could keep up the pace. Quite simply I wasn't taking care of myself.

Simonton asked, "Why did you do all these things? Couldn't you delegate?"

I replied, "Oh, no. It had to be me."

He said, "What if something happens to you? Who will do it then? If you die, do you think these things won't be done?"

I looked at him and said, "Yes, they'd get done without me. Not the same way, but yes, they would get done."

Dr. Simonton then said, "I'm telling you you are living a very unhealthful life-style. If you don't change it and start honoring yourself and taking care of your needs, you will die."

I somehow brushed aside this remark. I wouldn't listen. I backtracked to how much I was needed, to how it had to be me who took my daughter to the horse shows and drove Katrina to ballet class and flew to Canada when my brother was ill and again to London when my father was stricken. It *had* to be me who personally supervised every detail of running the houses, both here and in Vermont. It had to be me who supervised the horse business.

He put up his hand and stopped me in midflight. "You're not listening to me. If you don't stop and find time to change, you will die."

I said, "You don't understand. I can't help it."

Here Paul interrupted. "Mother, you don't know how to say no. If somebody calls and says, 'Can I leave my children with you while I take a vacation,' you don't want to do it. You know it will add stress to you, but you do it anyway."

I knew what he was referring to. I had agreed to take a friend's two children for the next ten days while they took a much-needed vacation. I immediately began my rebuttal.

"But, Paul, if I didn't who would?"

Dr. Simonton said, "I think you should listen to your son. He's trying to help you. It's clear to me that you are in an unhealthful situation. You must find a way to say no. You need peace and tranquility to get well."

I smiled, even found it humorous. He clearly didn't understand how needed I was. It would be many weeks before I fully understood what he was saying.

He then gave me a notepad and some colored crayons, telling me to draw a picture of myself. I drew a full figure, choosing a pink, flesh-colored crayon. I didn't bother to put clothes on it. However, in the hand of what resembled a cut-out paper doll, I drew with great detail in black crayon a basket, filling it with red cherries. With a blue crayon I gave myself eyes and with one stroke of a red crayon gave myself a faintly smiling mouth. I took a yellow crayon, and a few squiggles completed the portrait.

Paul sat in a corner. He was ready with the tape recorder. He would tape my first meditation.

Dr. Simonton solemnly studied my sketch.

"It's very interesting," he said, "but you have not detailed any part of your body or bothered to put clothes on it. However, you took great pains to draw the basket full of the red things."

He returned the portrait and asked me to choose any color to draw the cancer in my body. I chose a black crayon to make some random dots in the midsection of the form. Dr. Simonton looked at me.

"I think you see cancer as a powerful, dangerous, cunning disease, very difficult to get rid of. It is, in fact, a very weak disease composed of weak, confused, deformed cells. Its power is the rapidity with which it can grow, multiply and mutate."

In saying this, Dr. Simonton made his first step toward changing my basic beliefs about this devastatingly intimidating disease.

He turned to Paul and said, "If you are ready, I would like you to record the following meditation."

Then turning to me, "If you have to go to the bathroom, go now. I will require you to meditate for fifteen minutes and I would like you to be completely comfortable."

I took advantage of his invitation. I was so happy, happier than I had been since the onset of my illness. Here was someone who was going to teach me how to help myself.

It began this way with Dr. Simonton's voice:

Relax yourself. Physically relax yourself. I like to focus on my breathing, saying, "In" as I breathe in and "Out" as I breathe out. Being able to relax in the face of fear is incredibly powerful and very healthful. Now relax once more, deep relaxation. Now let's very simply go into thinking about cancer, moving very gently into that, specifically focusing upon cancer being a weak disease and the cancer cell being a weak, confused, deformed cell. And as it takes energy to push that belief in that direction, make a fist right now and think about cancer being a weak disease. Think about it being a weak disease composed of weak, confused, deformed cells and relax your fist.

And now think of chemotherapy coming into your body as your friend, helping you get rid of these cancer cells that are in your body and aligning yourself with it, such as you put rat poison in your house to help you get rid of rats, you don't go and eat the rat poison. Give your cells, your body, this kind of intelligence, this kind of energy, to increase their appreciation of what it is that you're doing. The purpose of the chemotherapy is to help your body get rid of any cancer cells. You're doing it for the good of your body, just as you put rat poison out for the good of your home and, as you think about your cells being smart and appreciating what you're doing in an attempt to improve your situation, make a fist.

Draw on that power and think about your being intelligent and understanding what you're doing and your cells being intelligent. They're part of you. And this making of the fist is adding energy to you to see it more vividly, to think about it more vividly. Then relax your fist.

Now think about your body's white blood cells. This is your representation really of you, and begin to think about your white blood cells doing the job that they're intended to do. Just as the wave does what it is intended to do, what it has done for millions of years, your white blood cells are doing what they have been programmed to do, what is built into them to do. You need to supply them with energy, so think about them going around taking care of your body. I want you to appreciate that and think about them. If they see any cancer cells, they destroy them. It's that simple, because that is what they're built to do, and you make a fist at this point, giving them the energy. They need energy. And so you're giving them the energy to do what they know how to do. You don't need to teach them anything. You need to supply them with some good energy. Think about them going along doing their job very competently, very potently, then just relax your fist.

And now, think about your life going in the direction you want it to go. Just the idea and the universe helping you, helping your life. You don't have to figure it out. You do what makes sense to you and open yourself to help. The wave doesn't sit around trying to figure out which is the shore. You don't need to figure out the direction of your life. You do what you understand to do, and you open yourself to help. The universe wants your life to go in its appropriate direction. The universe wants you to be healthy. The universe wants you to be happy. You open yourself to help, and the help will come; and that's something you need to practice. Merely by opening yourself to help and asking for it and waiting for it as you do what you understand to do.

I came out of the meditation and looked gratefully at Dr. Simonton. It was as if a dark cloud had been vacuumed away from around my head. Somehow this bear of a man had inspired me with the confidence to attack this disease, to hit it running. He wished me luck and I climbed back into the truck with Paul and he drove me home, with the precious meditation tapes, which were the beginning of my emotional healing.

Physically, I was already healing well. In Mitchell Karlan's absence, Dr. Uyeda removed the small metal stitches from my incision a few at a time with no discomfort. My arm was moving well and I had asked where I could buy a prosthesis. I wore my bikini swimsuits to sit in the sun with a silk scarf arranged in the right cup of my bra, but it was time to find something a bit more realistic.

Mitch's nurse sent me to a shop, Nearly Me, that specialized in prostheses. I sat on a pearl gray velvet couch, which looked as if it had been designed for a 1930s movie. I was nervous, embarrassed and a bit excited, looking forward to getting my new breast. I needed it; none of my clothes looked right.

But as I waited, surrounded by framed photographs of happy, smiling women, clad in bathing suits, all proudly throwing out their Nearly Me chests, I felt exposed and vulnerable. The young receptionist studied me curiously. I shifted in my seat, hoping she didn't recognize me. Fifteen minutes went by while I sat in the fancy false-tit shop. Finally, a middle-aged, ordinary-looking woman introduced herself as a trained prosthesis fitter. She took me to a dressing room.

"When did you have your surgery, and what size bra do you wear?" she asked.

"June second. Thirty-four B."

"Well, you may not be healed enough to wear the proper silicone breast form. We'll try the softer version. We call it the rest breast. Try this on." She handed me a bra.

I reluctantly removed my shirt. She stared at the scar. She was the first person apart from my surgeon and Charlie to see it. I was exposed, naked in a way I'd never felt before.

"Oh, you're still red and puffy. You're not ready for a proper prosthesis, but maybe you'll be able to wear the rest breast. Who's your surgeon? He did a really good job."

I gave her Mitchell Karlan's name and phone number. She said she often asked the names of good surgeons. She left the room and returned with a pink sponge-filled breast form. It was light in weight. She said it had to be inserted properly and asked me to lean forward so she could insert the form into the right cup. Then she gave the whole thing a yank and a shake.

"YEOW!" It hurt. Oh, God, I was still sore.

"Oh, I'm sorry, dear. Yes, you're still too tender for the heavier breast. Wait a minute, I want to get you a shirt so you can see how you'll look. Most women are thrilled when they see they can wear sheer fabrics."

She hurried out and returned with a silk shirt, obviously much used. It smelled of stale perspiration. I put it on, then studied myself. It was true, the silk lay over my breasts smoothly. I looked restored. No one would know anything. I took off the shirt and bra. I gave her the breast.

"I'll take one," I said as I put on my own comfortable, baggy shirt. I opened my purse and produced my charge card. She read it and turned her eyes to me.

Piercingly, "This card says Jill Ireland."

"Oh, yes, the card is still in my maiden name."

"Are you . . . are you the actress? The one that's married to Charles Bronson?"

"Yes, I am."

She looked at me accusingly. "Well, why don't you look the way you do on TV?"

Did she think I was an imposter? "Maybe you've been watching old movies. I'm older now, and I've just been through rather an ordeal." I wanted to get out of there. I was sick from fatigue and humiliation.

But she continued. "Oh, my, your husband is Charles

Bronson." She looked me up and down, relishing the moment. "How is he taking all this?"

I couldn't stand much more. Also, my chest hurt from the unaccustomed action. "He's fine, thank you."

"That's wonderful. You're so lucky, you know. I had a woman in here last week whose husband hasn't touched her since her mastectomy. He said she looked disgusting and that she disgusted him. The poor woman was completely demoralized."

A cold stream of perspiration trickled down under my arm. "Could you let me sign my charge now, please. I'm in a bit of a hurry." I needed to get away. I felt weak.

"Charles Bronson's wife. I can't believe it."

She stared hard over the top of her glasses. "Well, dear, you come back when you're ready to fit your proper prosthesis. This will do you for now, but the silicone form is more realistic. It has weight and won't ride up."

Shaky and light-headed, I took the charge card, signed the slip and left as fast as I could. I never went back. I sent my secretary to pick up the next breast I purchased. I considered myself a strong woman, sure of myself. What would have been her effect on a less secure person?

In spite of my experience at Nearly Me, I was grateful for the breast form. My chest did become sore from the pressure in the beginning. Also, if I wasn't careful, my new right breast had a tendency to pop out the top of my bra. I decided a couple of weeks later to get a thirty-three B form. The thirty-four B was bigger than my left breast in my swimsuits. I liked tightly stretched tank suits that year. They tended to flatten one's breasts. The smaller form matched better. Unless I raised my right arm to reveal the deep scar in my armpit, no one would know my secret. I was living at the beach house now and I had a deep tan. My hair had bleached to a pale blond and, so far, it hadn't fallen out. I'd been told I would begin losing it, but so far, so good.

At times I almost forgot living with cancer. We spent an evening watching the Democratic National Convention with

68

friends. But as soon as the television set was turned off and the good-nights said, I found myself wondering, *Why do I have this heavy feeling?* I'd soon remember. Or I'd wake up in the morning after a good night's sleep, wondering, *Why do I feel this way?* Did I have a nightmare last night? Then I remembered. It is a living, wide-awake nightmare. Ray Weston, whose first wife died of cancer, said it. "It's a fucking nightmare, Jill, a fucking nightmare."

In spite of all this, it was harder on my family than it was on me. Somewhere deep inside, I was grateful it was not so bad. I could still handle it. It could always get worse.

Then exactly two weeks after my first chemotherapy, I took a shower and whole handfuls of hair came out. I had stepped into the shower, relaxed and happy, turned on the water, and lathered up my head with shampoo. I rubbed my head vigorously, deep in thought. I sang as the water rinsed off the shampoo and fifty percent of my hair. My heart stopped. Great bird's nests of hair were all over the shower floor. I leaned against the tiled wall, trying to steady the pounding of my heart. The water poured down around me, filling the space with sound, but it was as if I were engulfed in silence. I could hear only my heart and thoughts. It started just as Michael said it would, just as I had always heard it did with chemotherapy. In every catastrophic event there is a single moment that makes it utterly real. Up until this moment in the shower, I knew I had cancer. I knew I was having chemotherapy. I knew I could die. But when I saw my hair lying around my ankles, my situation was suddenly brought home to me, for the first time.

I toweled myself dry and got ready to go to Michael's. Putting on the telltale mark of the female chemotherapy patient, I knotted a scarf over my head and Charlie and I set out for Michael's office, where we waited for the results of my white cell count. The count had been down the week before. Michael said there was a fifty-fifty chance I would receive my therapy that day. Charlie, desperately homesick for the farm, planned to leave for Vermont on Friday. I would have plenty of time to get over any sickness before he left. However, if I didn't get the therapy that day, he would be unable to leave until later. Charlie didn't look too pleased. He paced the small room, shoulders hunched. He was pent-up, trapped, suspicious of my doctor, angry at the illness that was changing and manipulating our lives.

Soon Michael came in. "It's okay, we do it."

"Good," said Charlie.

"Uh-oh," I said. In came the ice helmet and on went the tourniquet. I waited until my head was chilled, then onto the table I went. In came Michael. In went the needle. In went the first vial. Okay? Okay. I was chatting with the nurse. She actually took over and applied the Adriamycin slowly, more slowly than the last time. I felt nothing. Soon it was over. A further five minutes in the ice helmet, then back to the beach house.

That night I ate a light dinner and went to bed early. I awoke feeling okay. I vomited when I cleaned my teeth but, God, I felt okay. Later in the day I took a three-mile walk. I felt terrific. Hurray! I did it — all without antinausea drugs. Could it have been the meditation tape I had recorded and played to myself before I left for Michael's office?

I had some control over my body at last. "I feel terrific," I said. I didn't know that Michael had reduced the drugs for this second treatment.

I meditated three times a day as Dr. Simonton had instructed. I studied his book, *Getting Well Again,* carefully. His work to correct emotional attitudes about cancer had started to take hold.

"The cancer cell is a weak, confused cell," he had told me. "Your white blood cells are strong; your body has the power to heal itself." It was part of my meditation tape. I listened to it every day, even though some days I was too upset to concentrate as hard as I would have liked.

I rediscovered my love for the sea. It was now the most important element in my meditation and mental imagery. Instinct led me to spend my meditation hours by the ocean. I recorded the sound of the waves. I took walks along the beach with my German shepherd, Cassie.

The surging power of the ocean, wave after wave pounding the beach, reminded me of the power of the universe. There was a force stronger than myself, stronger than the minute cells waging a war within me. I wanted to tap into the mighty Pacific to absorb the ocean's energy and power, to make it part of me. I would walk to a giant rock and wait, counting the waves until the largest one would crash and spray over it. I looked for symbols everywhere. One day, walking on the beach, I came across a large balloon that somehow had escaped from a children's beach party. Immediately it became a perfect symbol for a cancer cell. Cassie was given the role of my white blood cells.

I pointed to the balloon. "Get it, Cassie. Kill it!"

In an instant, she pounced on the balloon and exploded it with a growl and snarl, ripping the rubber to shreds. This excited me. I used it many times in my mental visualization.

Charlie didn't quite share my love for the beach. He loved the trees in Vermont. His affinity was with them and their strength. Intellectually, I understood how much he needed to be there for himself and his own health. I wanted him to go, as I needed to prove to myself I could survive on my own. But I had mixed emotions.

"Go," I would say. "I'll be fine. Paul and Cassie will stay with me."

But at the same time, inside me, a little girl was saying, "Stay. I'll be scared — I need you. I feel sick and puny."

The week passed. I was fine. Friday came. Charlie and Zuleika left, and Paul moved into the beach house with me. Toward evening I began to feel ill. I called Ray.

"I feel strange, Ray. I'm sick."

He listened. "Well, dear, I'm here. Call me if you feel worse."

I went to bed about eleven and awoke at one, dreaming I was biting something as hard as I could. I was angry at it. It was hurting me. I sobbed myself awake.

The next night I awoke again at one. This time I was being attacked by an angry cat. It would hurl itself on my right arm, scratching and clawing at me. I would fling it off, and it would fly back at me again. I awoke screaming.

The next day I was exhausted and in the evening I was ill again. I had the sensation of having been given an anesthetic. There was the vague onion taste in my throat, and my legs were shaking. I thought I was going to pass out. Paul called my doctors. No one home. God. We finally contacted a stand-in for Michael. He thought I was having an anxiety attack, or perhaps my white blood cells had dropped below comfort level.

"Take a Valium and call me in the morning."

Shit. I can't believe it. Ray called back.

"What is it, dear? No, you're not a nuisance."

I described my feelings. He also prescribed Valium plus an antacid. I hung up, took a Dalmane, four antacids and lay in bed talking to Paul. I thought things over. Is it possible I am so anxious it's making me sick? Could this awful physical sensation be coming from inner emotion? Okay, I would find out. Tomorrow I would phone a holistic counselor.

I recalled my dream. What did the cat want? Could it be my inner self demanding I pay attention to parts of me I hadn't been honoring for a long time? If my emotions could make me sick, surely I could use my emotions to make myself well. I went to sleep holding this thought, and slept without nightmares.

12

I MADE AN APPOINTMENT with a woman trained in holistic healing and meditation. I'd been told she knew about Dr. Simonton's techniques. A friend of mine, a makeup artist, had been treated by her for two years. Alan, dear Alan, slick, street-smart, raised in an English working-class mill town, Alan Marshall had been my friend for twenty years.

We never stayed down for long; we loved to laugh too much. Our relationship had survived my first marriage, my divorce and remarriage. Alan was close to all my children, and he admired, almost revered, Charlie. Because of his tremendous respect for Charlie, he had applauded and supported my decision to marry him, making the observation, "Although you are complete opposites, I think he's perfect for you."

Alan's behavior was often outrageous, but to me he was always loving and giving. Since my surgery, he had tried to convince me to see Sue Colin, but I had resisted. I wasn't ready. But now my scar was healed; my energy was up. It was time for me to discover why I had become sick. Medical science helped and was doing its best. But I knew that the next and perhaps most important part was up to me.

The day came. Alan, sweet soul, drove a long distance to take me for my first visit. He said repeatedly he knew Sue Colin was going to help. On her door it said, SUE COLIN, M.A., HOLISTIC COUNSELING CENTER. I went in.

The medical profession gives you a double message. Doctors

recite statistics and facts. Then they cut off pieces, give you chemotherapy and afterward send you home, advising you to have a positive attitude — "everything will be fine." It is almost impossible to keep a positive attitude on your own. The fear is so all-consuming, the loneliness so vast. A self-searching exploration with a counselor or therapist can be a vital part of recovery and learning to live with cancer.

So I began the hard work of self-discovery.

Sue Colin is an attractive, warm woman, an Earth Mother, with a lusty zest for life. She is about my age, with dark hair and brown eyes. She was to start me off this day on my journey into self. I had no trouble talking to her. It was a relief to be able to talk freely about my illness, about my fears. I couldn't talk to Charlie about them. He would retreat from the subject. He resented cancer conversations. It was as if he feared he would catch the cancer if he identified with me. He loved me, but he simply didn't want to listen.

So I told Sue Colin about the stresses leading up to my surgery and the different people in my life. I discussed my feelings about surgery and the loss of my breast. I told her the surgery was really not so bad, and I was adjusting well to the loss of my right breast and the loss of my hair. I talked about my husband and daughter being away for two weeks, how I felt the need to be alone, even though I was scared. I talked and talked for an hour and a half. It was as if deep inside me a fist were unclenching.

During the first week I saw Sue every day and thereafter three times a week. With the help of meditation, I regressed in my memory to the despair and grief I felt as a baby of ten months when I had Pinkus' disease, a disease of the blood, which necessitated my mother's leaving me in a hospital for some months. I was put in a glass incubator in isolation. When she visited, I would cry and hold out my arms to her, but she wasn't allowed to hold me. Her visits upset me so much she stopped coming. With Sue to guide me, I meditated and actually saw a little girl in a glass case sitting in diapers looking out at me — not crying — just sitting quietly.

74

As the picture came to me, I fought back sadness and a desire to weep. She told me to ask the child what she was feeling.

I replied, "She feels nothing."

Sue told me to pick up the baby and hold her. I put out my arms and placed the baby next to my breast, feeling the warm, relaxed baby form. As I held the little girl, I felt such a wave of compassion and sorrow that I burst out sobbing. Then I became quiet.

Sue told me, "When you think she's been held long enough, tell her you are sorry you left her and you will never leave her again. Then take the little girl into your body and feel her warmth inside you. Tell her you will be there to hold her whenever she needs it."

I did all this, feeling deeply satisfied, relaxed and complete. We finished the meditation and I opened my eyes. It was a major breakthrough for me. And I was to have many more.

One of the most important thresholds I crossed was discussing my anxiety attacks. I had been subject to them for most of my life. They manifested themselves by generally impeding my ability to breathe or swallow. They began as far back as my nervous sniffing as a child and reappeared in the form of hyperventilating in my adult life. Sue asked me to meditate. As I did, once more I felt myself pushing back the desire to cry when asked to confront my anxiety. She asked me to induce an attack. I was scared and reluctant. I always thought anxiety was going to kill me, that I would freeze up, choke and stop breathing. I let the throat constrictions start. I became frightened as my breathing became more difficult. Then Sue asked what I was afraid of.

"I don't want to die. I don't want to leave Zuleika and Charlie." I was racked with sorrow, anger and the raw fear of death. Sue sat quietly beside me until it was over and I felt calm again. I had confronted my fears. Now I hoped the anxiety attacks would stop.

On Alan's recommendation, I also began seeing Bernard Dowson, a homeopathic doctor. Homeopathy was new to me, but I knew the royal family of England had for many years employed homeopathic doctors. Alan's nickname for me was "the Empress," so a homeopathic practitioner seemed appropriate.

Homeopathic medicine involves the ancient art of using nature's elements, herbs and minerals, and in some cases harnessing electrical currents to help effect health. Since my frustrating experience with the nonunion of my right ankle bone, which stubbornly refused to heal until the electromagnetic impulse machine was used on it, I had had faith in electromagnetic medicine, so homeopathy was not so strange to me as it might have been.

Bernard Dowson told me, "What I do is make your body stronger, healthier, more in balance. I let your body worry about illnesses if they exist. The immune system has very sophisticated antibodies that can kill any abnormality. Your body has that incredible intelligence. My feeling is that cancer develops when your body is in a weakened condition. Everyone has cancer cells. You allowed some of them to grow."

I asked Bernard to tell me more about the process. He said, "A medical team in Sweden has completed a clinical study of electronic, low-frequency magnetic wave tables with a high success rate in the treatment of cancer. In Russia, three different groups of physicists are using magnetic tables to cure cancer, and they say they don't know why it works, but it does. Tumors go away. Just with this kind of device."

Had I got to such a point that I was prepared to go for these taken-on-faith-only cures? Was I operating from a position of fear or was I perhaps pioneering? I talked to Michael Van Scoy Mosher about it.

He said, "The trouble with these sorts of methods is that they rely on all kinds of tests that no one but the practitioner can understand, so there is no way to prove it out. However, I don't think it can hurt you, Jill. And it may help."

If Bernard Dowson could help me, I was going to give him every opportunity to do so.

Bernard gave me small bottles of a remedy that had been electrically charged. I drank the potion eight times a day.

Twice a week, I lay on a table he had designed with electromagnetic wave vibrations to rebalance my body's cells. During our first meeting, Bernard took a saliva test and a snip of my hair. He also put an electrical acupuncture device on my right ear. He told me my vitality and energy potential was high and that I should have no trouble getting well, but I should probably get some therapy to help me handle the fear I was experiencing. I told Bernard that Sue Colin was already fulfilling that mission.

I meditated three times a day religiously; it gave me a task, something I could do alone to get myself well. I was given back some control over my destiny. I recalled the moment when I learned I had cancer. At the instant I had heard those fateful words, something in me had kicked over. It was as if a switch had been thrown. I felt myself gather all my forces and begin to fight. The energy was there waiting to be tapped. It knew what to fight. The enemy was within my body. The question was how.

Now I had the ammunition I needed in my war against cancer. The AMA had done its part in amputating my breast and scheduling chemotherapy every three weeks. For that elusive "good attitude," I was learning to look to homeopathic medicine and holistic healing to guide and encourage me on the long voyage to health.

Drowning in an uncharted sea, I gathered bits of driftwood, piece by piece, linking them together until they became a life raft to help keep me afloat through the calms, swells and storms that would befall me in the coming months.

Meditation helped me visualize the white blood cells destroying my cancer and was a means of relieving stress and quieting my mind.

I also grasped the healing properties of quartz crystals for focusing and energizing my mind and body. A crystal is the only thing in the world that has a perfect molecular order; it is, in fact, perfect order. Sue Colin used them for healing. She would hold a crystal in her hand, drawing the healing energy into her. Sometimes when I was with her, I would meditate using the energy of the crystal. I began collecting crystals. I had a large amethyst crystal, small crystal clusters and one beautiful large crystal wand. I held them during my cancer meditation. I wore a crystal close to my throat on a chain around my neck. I hung another over my heart. I kept three on the bedside table and one large cluster on the coffee table in the sitting room. They were certainly beautiful and I enjoyed looking at them.

With Charlie away for a couple of weeks, I had been forced to turn inward for emotional support. This was good. I was getting used to being without him and Zuleika. Any instinct to cling to Charlie as my savior had been put aside.

"Okay, kid," I told myself, "you're on your own. Michael Van Scoy Mosher will do his best. The rest is up to you. Go out there, try anything. You have nothing to lose but cancer."

The phone rang, making me jump. I got up from the deep wicker-basket couch with its oatmeal linen cushions. I took the phone to the veranda to watch the ocean as I talked. It was Lesley-Anne Down, the beautiful British actress who had become popular in America in the television series "Upstairs, Downstairs." She was married to film director William Friedkin, our next-door neighbor in Bel Air for many years, who had come into prominence with the terrifying film *The Exorcist*. They had a lovely blue-eyed, blond baby boy they called Jack.

Jason had kept up his acquaintance with Billy Friedkin and was now good friends with Angela Down, Lesley-Anne's younger sister. But I was surprised to hear from Lesley because we really didn't socialize much. Her rich, plummy English accent tickled my ears and my sense of humor.

"Dahling, how are you?" she greeted me on the telephone. "Jason told me you've rented a beach house for the summer."

"Well," she went on, "we've rented a house in the Malibu

Colony." Lesley's voice drawled on like an English Tallulah Bankhead, "Dahling, I'm giving a luncheon."

The word *luncheon* became a feast in itself, and having pronounced it, Lesley needed a second or two to digest it.

"Yes, dahling, a small, intimate luncheon for just a few people. I would love it if you and Charlie could come."

"Well, Charlie's in Vermont and I haven't been going out much lately."

"Oh I know, dahling, but do come if you feel up to it. Bring anyone you like. I would love to see you. Being a fellow English person and all, I'm sure we have things to say to each other — both being married to Americans and all that."

Here Lesley was distracted a moment. "Jack! Jack!" Lesley called into her house.

She came back to the phone and said, "Oh, excuse me. I've got to get Jack away from the bar. He's an alcoholic, dahling, he's always going behind the bar."

Lesley certainly had an amusing way of expressing herself. I laughed.

"My God, Lesley, I hope you can curtail this activity. How old is he now, anyway?"

"He's two, dahling. I've got to go now. Jack! Come here, dahling. See you on Sunday then. One-thirty. Bye. Do come, I'd love it."

She hung up to more cries of "Jack! Put that down."

Well, I thought it might be amusing. Paul could escort me. She said it would be a small group. It might be good for me.

On Sunday at one-forty-five, arriving fashionably fifteen minutes late, Paul, his girlfriend Priscilla and I rang the bell at the Friedkins' attactive beach house. From the street you would never suspect it was situated on the sand. The back of the house — or was it considered the front? — had a small garden hidden by a high, white-painted brick wall. The house was like a small country cottage, reminiscent of England. A buzz indicated the lock on the gate was unlatched, so we pushed the door and entered.

Inside, out of the bright sunlight, my first reaction was that we were all overdressed, me in my large pink straw hat with roses covering the brim and my pale pink cotton minidress and delicate strappy sandals with little silk flowers entwined around the straps. Priscilla was in a dress and Paul wore his customary outfit: shorts, cotton shirt and sandals. Standing before a long table spread with food was what appeared to be — since she had her back to the light — a naked lady, a very brown naked lady. Beside her was a small, brown, naked two-year-old boy. The sight startled me as I suspect it did Paul and Priscilla. Then the lady spoke and moved toward us.

"Dahling," said the now-familiar voice of Lesley-Anne, "I'm so glad you could make it."

As she moved toward us I saw that my first impression was an error, but only by a slim margin. She was wearing three triangles, very small ones. Two tiny pieces of cloth over her breasts and a minuscule triangle over her lower parts. Her body was in superb shape. Her blond hair had been pulled back simply and her tanned face was free of makeup. Looking out of all this bronzed skin were a pair of large, pale blue eyes. Lesley looked magnificent and I told her as much.

"Thank you, dahling. Would you like to borrow a bathing suit?"

I had to smile at her old-fashioned term for what she was wearing.

"Oh, no thank you, at least not one of yours, wonderful though it looks on you."

Lesley turned, giving me the chance to see that the designer had run out of material for the back of her bathing suit and had satisfied himself by simply running a thong up the back that disappeared between her muscular buttocks. Wow! It was a wondrous sight.

"William's around somewhere. He's the bartender. Help yourself to food."

Little Jack Friedkin was indeed naked. He came to me happily, a most adorable little boy with blond curly hair and his mother's big blue eyes. He held his small penis in hand.

80

"Pee-pee," he said proudly, looking up at me.

I smiled at him. He reminded me of my own blond Valentine at that age.

"Yes, Jack, and it's a very nice one, too."

Jack responded in a typically masculine way to my compliment. He followed me outside to the patio, smiling, where to my surprise the small luncheon was much larger than I expected. Several important studio executives were there, and I noticed others dressed similarly to myself, I was glad to see. They all mixed and mingled in the bright sunlight. It was a pretty setting with the patio designed like an English garden, with flowers and a lawn that led to a deck overlooking the beach and the ocean.

Jack followed me to the deck. It seemed I had made a conquest. On the way Jack stopped several times, said, "Pee-pee," and did just that wherever he stood. He was obviously accustomed to wearing diapers and so relieved himself wherever and whenever he felt like it. It didn't help matters that he picked up guests' drinks and guzzled them with a baby's urgency as the hot sun beat down on his little head.

I remembered my own small boys and how I had toilet trained them in the summer. I had, like Lesley, allowed them to run around naked in the sunshine. Then whenever they needed to urinate, I had told them to water the flowers, taking them over to my camellia plants. They watered the flowers and learned control as they saved themselves for the flourishing blossoms. I decided to try this on Jack. His little belly was round and distended from all the drinks he had been pilfering from his parents' guests.

Now he returned to my side where I was sitting with Paul on the deck. He picked up my orange juice and drank deeply.

"Jack," I said. "When you have to go pee-pee I want you to do it on the flowers."

"Pee-pee," said Jack. "Flowers?"

"Yes, sweetheart, pee-pee on the flowers."

Jack ran off in search of more orange juice, probably. I was not feeling outgoing and gregarious and no one was particularly anxious to make my acquaintance — perhaps they felt uncomfortable about my illness — although I did know many of the guests. But I was happy sitting on the chair by the beach. I always enjoyed people-watching and from under the low brim of my hat, my eyes concealed by dark glasses, I could watch undetected and unashamedly. In a short while Jack returned.

"Pee-pee," he said, carefully thrusting his little belly toward me. Then he peed all over my legs and feet.

I was amazed and speechless. Paul burst out laughing.

"Well, Mother, you did tell him to pee-pee on the flowers."

I looked down. There, sure enough, glistening after their bath, were the pert flowers on my sandals. Jack had, with the precision of a child's observation, noticed them on my arrival and happily obliged me when I suggested he pee-pee on the flowers. He was now mopping my legs with a paper serviette.

"Oh, Jack," I said, giving him a hug. "You are such a good boy."

I sat him on my knee and saw that he was getting sleepy. Lesley came by.

"Come on, Jack. It's time for your nap."

She retrieved her now half-asleep son. A nanny appeared with a baby bottle and the last I saw of Jack he was being carried away happily drinking. It occurred to me that some of what Jack had been imbibing during the afternoon may have been alcoholic and that Jack would probably sleep long and hard as a result. I remembered Lesley's words on the phone, *He's an alcoholic, dahling*. I felt suddenly tired and sad. I wanted to go home. I told Paul and Priscilla I would walk the two and a half miles along the beach to our house. So I jumped off the deck and struck out for home with my wet sandals in my hand. I had had more than enough socializing for one day.

13

THE TWO WEEKS HAD now passed. Charlie and Zuleika were due home from Vermont in time for my third chemotherapy. Earlier I had telephoned Charlie to tell him I was doing fine without him and Zuleika and that they should remain in Vermont.

"Stay there," I urged. "Darling, truly, I'm fine. I want you and Zuleika to stay there as long as you want. Please, I don't need you."

"That's nice, Jill, but I'm coming home. It's enough. I miss you and I'm coming home."

I was secretly happy. I'd be glad to see Charlie, and I'd missed Zuleika tremendously. But I was also pleased to know I had been telling the truth, that I didn't need them to come home, even though I hated the thought of chemo more than before. Chemo makes you feel as if it is going to kill you. You literally feel you are dying. Every part of you is warning, *Don't take any more. The next time it will kill you.*

I sat in Michael's office once more, waiting for the results of my blood test. I knew from my mental imagery while meditating that the white cells were handling the chemotherapy all right. I would have been surprised if my white cell count was down. It wasn't. I tried to relax as I sat wearing the ice helmet.

In came Michael. Off we went again. In went the needle and the white 5FU. Everything was okay. Then in went the

Adriamycin, and suddenly I felt it, a burning all over my body. My veins felt full to bursting. Every instinct in my body screamed, *Stop, you got away with it the last time, but stop now. It's going to kill you.*

I couldn't stand it. I asked Michael to stop. He said he was nearly finished, that he wouldn't be doing me a favor if he stopped. I wanted to rip the needle out of my arm and run far away. I hung on. When it was over, I lay on the table, weak, already nauseated, waves of sickness shooting through me. I knew there was nothing anyone could do. I would just have to put up with it.

I somehow returned to the beach house. The rest of the long night I was sick. It was much worse than the first two treatments. I suspected I had been given a heavier dose of drugs. I went to bed but couldn't sleep. I just lay there thinking of an expression I'd heard once, "Oh, Lord, you made the night too long."

I struggled through the next day. Alan came to take me to see Bernard Dowson. I lay on the electromagnetic table in an enclosed cubicle, feverish and nauseated. I tried to meditate, but I was hot and miserable. Suddenly the curtains parted and in came Sue Colin. She was there to have a table treatment herself. Saying she was sorry I was so sick, Sue put her arms around me. She held me for a few minutes, then putting a beautiful piece of rock crystal in my hand, she left. I began to cry. It was a relief to feel sad and sorry for myself. Holding on to the quartz, experiencing the relief and healing power of tears, I realized I had been fighting compassion for myself. It took Sue's motherliness and warmth to allow me to get in touch with it. It was okay to feel sorry for myself.

I lay on the table for an hour listening to the music that always played when I took the treatment. I wondered why I never felt anything, not even a tingle. But then I remembered the electromagnetic impulse machine strapped to my ankle with the current going through my broken bone; I hadn't felt anything then either. Maybe the table was doing its work after all. By the time Margaret, Bernard's sweet receptionist, came to get me, I was feeling better. I don't know if it was the table, Sue or time, but I did feel better.

The third chemo, though, brought a new turn of events. Eleven days after that treatment, white, painful lumps appeared in my mouth, on my tongue and in my throat. It became almost impossible to eat or drink. Even water passing over the affected areas caused terrible pain. My bottom lip was swollen and sore. Michael said it was a rare reaction to chemotherapy. As he put it, the white lumps were evidence that I had reached my full capacity. He said he would cut down the potency on the fourth chemotherapy. I felt somewhat relieved, but worried it might mean I would have to continue longer with treatments. Michael assured me that would not be the case. I was almost grateful for the hideous mouth sores if they meant the chemo would be diluted. The sores lingered twelve days. During that time I lost a great deal of weight. Charlie watched helplessly as I dropped pounds. He looked so sad. He was still having trouble accepting the reality of my condition. I would catch him staring at me. I knew I was losing my appearance. I knew I looked ill.

In other respects I felt good. My energy level was up, and I started riding my horses again. Slowly and carefully, to be sure, but I was riding. My prosthesis was convincing, except when I rode. Then only one breast bounced; the other stayed steadfastly looking straight ahead. Once during my aerobic exercise class my right breast rotated until it was upside down. Worse, it began to work its way out of the top of my leotard. I didn't discover what was happening until it was too late and the prosthesis bounced on the floor among the other exercisers. After that experience, I pinned it inside my bra. In all other ways, I wore the same clothes as before, except for deep décolletage.

By now, I had a large collection of hats — small porkpies, boaters and large, romantic straws. My hair was extraordinarily thin, and I didn't like to be seen without a hat. I had a large bald spot on the crown of my head.

About this time, I received a visit from my dear, if some-

85

what eccentric, friend Marcia Borie. Witty, intelligent, highly successful, Marcia is editor of the *Hollywood Reporter*. I love her sense of humor and ability to laugh at herself. We go back a long way. I hadn't seen her since I became ill. Concerned that I was perhaps dying, she drove from her San Fernando Valley home to spend the day with me. I was sure she dreaded seeing me, imagining the worst. Her mother had died of cancer when she was a young girl. To spare her the sight of my wispy, thinning hair, I selected a bright Mexican cotton scarf and tied it gypsy fashion, with the knot on the side of my head for added dash.

I found myself looking forward to Marcia's visit. She arrived all a-bustle, bearing gifts — small, prettily wrapped packages of tea, bath beads, jams and candles from England, things she knew I liked. For the first time in our relationship, we were awkward with each other. I wanted to see her, but not this way, in the role of cancer victim. To ease the awkwardness, I suggested a walk on the beach. She changed into shorts and a T-shirt, and off we went down the strand with Cassie. We spoke of the beautiful day, the blue of the sea, both of us avoiding *the* conversation. I wasn't in the mood to discuss cancer. It was too exhausting. I wished we could just enjoy one another's company as if nothing had happened.

Suddenly, down the beach, running toward us, came a small, familiar figure. Cassie recognized him first. With a yelp of joy, she dashed off to meet Alan. Alan and Marcia hadn't seen each other for fourteen years.

"Marcia, you old sow bag," said Alan unceremoniously, "how are you? You look just the same."

Marcia received the greetings with equanimity and smiled. "My God, Alan, after all these years. You look wonderful."

I was pleased by Alan's unexpected visit. Things were more relaxed. We went into the house for lunch, where Paul joined us. We were a happy group, chatting and laughing as we ate our salads.

Alan left after lunch and Paul took his Windsurfer out on

the ocean, sailing far out until he was no more than a bright speck in the distance. Marcia sat beside me on the couch and we finally talked. It was so nice. We were Jill and Marcia again with no strains. Just two old friends. The time passed too quickly. Marcia had to leave. We hugged good-bye. It had turned out to be a good visit. I was pleased my scarf had ful-filled its purpose in concealing my sparse hair. Marcia had taken no note of it.

It was strange how whimsically selective the chemotherapy was when it came to burning out my hair. I had lost nearly all the hair on my head, all my pubic hair and some of the down on my arms. However, I still had my eyelashes and eyebrows and fuzz on my cheeks and chin, which Charlie called my whiskers. Also I still grew hair in my underarms.

This presented a problem since I had lost all feeling in my right armpit, making shaving it a difficult and hazardous un-dertaking. One would have thought I'd have been grateful for hair growing anywhere. But no, perversely, I wanted smooth underarms. I bought an electric razor but because I couldn't feel what I was doing, I always missed places, leaving behind small tufts, which frustrated me and offended my sense of personal order. Pinching and rubbing my numb skin heed-lessly, I would go over the area again and again, to no avail. Burr, buzz, buzz went my Lady Gillette, until I had sore red spots.

I was close to tears when Charlie walked into the bathroom we shared at the beach house. He saw my frustration. Gently, he took the shaver from my hand and carefully put talcum powder over the surgery scars in the area I had been mutilat-ing. Then with great concentration and tenderness he shaved me neatly. It was almost the nicest thing anyone had ever done for me.

My stepdaughter, Suzanne, telephoned to say she had heard of a doctor who gave chemotherapy without side effects. I called and asked Michael if he knew about a method of re-ceiving the drugs slowly once a week in weaker doses.

He said, "I don't know anything about it."

I pushed the idea from my mind until one night Charlie and I were invited to dinner with an ex-actress and her husband. She was a woman of perhaps fifty-eight, very feminine, looking much younger than her years. She had had breast cancer, then lung and throat cancer. We discussed the horror of chemotherapy. She said that after six months, she told her doctor, "Enough, I won't take any more. I can't stand another injection."

Then she mentioned she had completed eighteen months of chemotherapy with the doctor Suzanne had told me about — the one who applied the chemicals so slowly that there were no unpleasant aftereffects. She visited the doctor once a week and sat with other patients, chatting and reading magazines while an IV slowly dripped the drugs into her. She said her hair stopped falling out, she stopped feeling ill and even drove herself for treatments, going shopping afterward. Compared to what I was going through, it sounded like Xanadu.

Surely, Michael must know some doctors who administered the chemicals in that manner. I decided to tell him how I felt and to talk to Ray Weston about the other oncologist. Before I had the opportunity, I attended a horse show with Zuleika, and talked with Dr. Adler, the father of another young rider. I asked him about the doctor everyone had been telling me about. Dr. Adler said he knew the man. In fact, he used to send his patients to the doctor, but he believed I was getting my chemotherapy the right way. Dr. Adler said the other means was a very mild treatment. He knew I had had cancer on eight lymph nodes.

"You must get a fully loaded dose," he said.

It reminded me of Michael saying the blisters in my mouth were a good indication, indeed, that I had received a full dose.

When we got home that night, Ray called and spoke to Charlie. Charlie told him how I was progressing and mentioned the oncologist who gave weekly treatments. Ray knew the doctor. In fact, he had treated Ray's wife, but he didn't think his treatment was right for me, saying, "No, Jill, for you it's not the way to go."

Okay, so be it. I started to wind up my courage in preparation for Thursday's fourth chemo. I should have known better than to confuse myself with conflicting advice.

14

 A DOZEN WEEKS after surgery I mourned the loss of my breast.

I stood up in the tub after soaking in fragrant bath oil. I looked into the mirror across the room. My body was gleaming and tanned. I saw a pretty torso, small-waisted, narrow-hipped; my stomach was flat and smooth, free of stretch marks. I looked with almost narcissistic pleasure. I stood full figure in the mirror. In the steam of the bathroom, the image I saw looked like a shot from a girlie magazine, except it was a bizarre parody. This pinup model had only one breast. Everything else was the way I expected to see it, but the right side of my torso was flat, like a boy's, with a slash of a scar running across it. I looked for a long time, holding my left breast in my hand. I caressed it, trying to remember what it had been like to hold both breasts in my hands. I felt sad, sorry for my breast. I missed it and found myself wondering where it was, what they had done with it. I would like to have buried it. I mourned it like the loss of an old friend. For the first time I realized it was gone forever.

It had been a good friend. My children had slept on it, my husband had taken pleasure in it. It had been featured, bouncing merrily, in many bikinis, tank tops, leotards and teddies. It had made stately appearances from the top of evening gowns and had served me well. Poor thing. I hadn't even said good-bye. I had not seen it since the day of my biopsy. I wished I had cupped it in my hands one last time, my old friend, my right breast. All the years I had spent oiling and creaming it, doing exercises to keep it firm. Now, with one swift move, it was gone. Chop, chop. A little mastectomy with chemotherapy for dessert.

My friend Alan was the most positive influence anyone could wish. He couldn't imagine any future for me but total recovery. This meant no more chemo, no more cancer, complete hair regrowth and reconstructive surgery. He would say, "I can't wait, girl, till we get your tit put back. We'll find the best tit man in the business."

"Alan, there's no rush. I'm not ready. I have to earn my tits. I've got to shape up my thighs first."

"Well, get those thighs firmed up, girl, then it's off to the surgeon as soon as you've finished your chemo."

He cut my hair, artfully arranging the crown and sides, all the time hunting for regrowth. The wig I had had made looked wonderful, but so far I hadn't worn it. We even went so far as to have hair sewn into the bands of a couple of hats so my hair and hat went on and off in one move. I hadn't used the hats either. I was managing with scarves and my collection of straws. Charlie didn't want anyone to see my bald spots.

He said, "Babe, when this is all over, I don't want anyone to look at you and remember how you look now. Also, you want people to relate to you as Jill, not as someone to feel sorry for. Put your hat on."

So I always wore a hat or scarf over my head. If it had been left to me, I would have fluffed up the front pieces and walked on the beach as I was. I couldn't see the back of my head, so it didn't bother me. In my case, what the eye didn't see, the heart didn't grieve.

Later that day I took a walk and found myself wondering if the people I met knew about me. I saw Johnny Carson. I had been a guest on his show several times. He was walking with an attractive woman. He smiled, "Hello, how are you feeling?"

"I'm fine, how are you?"

I wondered if he knew. I suspected he did. It was weird.

The sea never failed to pick up my spirits and I spent many a day between chemo treatments poking around, looking for a beach house to buy. Now Charlie agreed that living at the beach was a pleasurable experience. One day we found a house we wanted to buy. It was much smaller than our Bel Air home. It was right on the ocean. It had been built in the thirties by Jack L. Warner, the founder of Warner Brothers Studios. It needed considerable work to restore its former glory. The prospect excited me, and I nicknamed the Spanish-Mediterranean property the House That Jack Built.

I loved this house. It was so compact. It had only three bedrooms upstairs. Perfect. One for me and Charlie, one for Zuleika and one for Katrina. All other members of the family still living at home would be given their eviction orders. The ground floor, once comprised of three small rooms, had been opened up by the removal of two walls and was now a single rambling living area overlooking the ocean. I liked the large, double-sided fireplace in the middle. The kitchen was big enough to accommodate a generous table and chairs, another bonus. My family and friends tend to congregate in the kitchen to socialize over a glass of wine, a cup of tea or a piece of cheesecake. Actually, some of the livelier conversations taking place in our home started around our butcher-block kitchen table.

In contrast to the Bel Air house, the beach house would give me the chance for a simpler life-style — fewer servants, fewer possessions, fewer responsibilities. I would be getting eight rooms in exchange for the twenty-three in Bel Air, four bathrooms instead of twelve, three telephones in place of twelve.

What would I do with all the antique Oriental rugs? This

house I saw with primitive Mexican handwoven rugs scattered on its tiled floors, bright touches in rooms where I would paint the walls white and bring the wood back to its natural hue. No more padded fabric and chintz walls, no more silk and damask antique chairs. Bye-bye two old friends, the oversized Queen Anne tapestry wingback chairs. I wondered what I would do with the rooms of furniture, paintings, silver and art objects. I thought about the silver candelabras and trays displayed in the dining room. They would have to go, as they would tarnish too quickly in the beach air. I would be trading my view of the rolling fairways and greens of the Bel Air Country Club for the nonstop moving entertainment of the beach and the rolling majesty of the Pacific Ocean. I was ready.

Thursday came, my fourth chemotherapy. Sue Colin had made a meditation tape for me. I planned to wear a headset under the ice helmet and meditate while Michael gave me the treatment. Time had dulled a lot of my fear.

I awoke early and took Zuleika to the barn to school her horse before the day became uncomfortably hot. We were suffering a heat wave with temperatures as high as one hundred and four. I was taking one day at a time, then narrowing it down to one moment at a time — living only in the moment. If that moment were pleasurable, causing no pain, I didn't think of past moments or future moments. This method helped fend off fear.

I derived tremendous pleasure watching my beautiful daughter ride in the morning sun. She was glowing, just beginning to mature physically. I looked at her small breasts, feeling a surge of love and compassion for her and all womankind.

After a light lunch, Charlie and I went straight to Michael's office. As I got out of the elevator and faced his office door, the cool, living-in-the-moment lady suddenly burst into tears and cowered in the corner, face to the wall. "I don't want to go in."

Poor Charlie. What could he do? "I wish I could take it for you." Charlie never says anything unless he means it. Hearing him say that meant so much to me.

I said sincerely, "Thank you, Charlie," wiped my eyes and went in.

After the blood test, Michael told me my first dose had been fully loaded, the second a bit less strong and the third a full dose. That explained the differences in my reactions. His nurse Michelle was a favorite of mine. I asked her to give me the injection, which she did while Michael stood beside me with Charlie.

Michael was interested in my meetings with Dr. Simonton, and his holistic medicine. He was particularly interested in my reaction to Simonton's admonition that I would die if I didn't change my way of life. I was already trying not to squander all my energy, but to use it on myself and self-healing. Michael told me he knew a Simonton patient who had been told the same thing. The patient had asked Simonton, "How do you know I'll die if I don't change my life-style?"

I didn't feel it appropriate to challenge Simonton. I went to him believing he knew. If your life-style makes you ill, then surely you can heal yourself with the right effort and thought.

Michelle completed my injection and applied the Band-Aid. She had injected the chemicals slowly; it was a lighter dose than the last, so I didn't experience burning or nausea. I sat up shakily and said good-bye to Michael.

Once home, I went immediately to the beach and stood in the ocean. The tide brought in some stones in shades of pink, pale blue and gray. I picked up four: two pink, one blue and a larger one with multicolored stripes of gray, pink and white. I put them on the coffee table to represent my four remaining chemo treatments. I was halfway through, halfway home.

The evening passed uneventfully. My only reaction was a bad lower back pain that spread down my legs. The pain was preferable to the awful nausea. The next day the temperature continued to climb all the way up the thermometer to one hundred and eleven. I lay around hot and listless, unable to distinguish between chemotherapy reaction and my response to the weather. Probably a bit of both. I lay listening to the ocean, contemplating the odds on full recovery. I rarely thought in those terms. When I did, my stomach dropped with an almost audible thud.

Nothing seemed to go well. We had made a bid on the Jack Warner house. The real estate broker called to say the bid, our limit, had been turned down. That was depressing. I was negotiating with my agent over a script I wanted to sell. He hadn't called, so that deal hadn't gone through. I was also discussing a role in a television show. I wanted to demonstrate to anyone who cared that I was full of zip and looking good (I planned to achieve this miracle with the wig, a makeup job by Alan and careful rationing of my energy). I didn't hear back. All these irons were no longer in the fire. I was left in the muggy heat only battling my disease.

I wandered onto the beach in my bikini without my hat, wanting to stand in the water and cool off. My hair was standing up, bald spots showing. I looked pale and tired; my body was small and thin. Charlie and Zuleika were lying together on an inner tube, looking fit and beautiful with their limbs gleaming in the water. I wondered what I was doing in such a healthy-looking family.

A man approached. It was Army Archerd, the writer from *Daily Variety*. He looked at me kindly.

"Hello, Jill. How are you?"

"Oh, I'm fine, Army, fine."

After all the trouble I had taken with hats and glasses, here I was unveiled, practically naked, talking to a reporter. He chatted with Charlie, who told him about my illness. I felt exposed, hot and uncomfortable.

That weekend was hard going. I had no appetite, no will to do anything. The toxicity was poisoning me and, hopefully, killing the cancer cells. All I could do was wait.

15

THE GIRLS' FALL SCHOOL semester started the next day. I braided Zuleika's hair and kissed both girls good-bye before sending them off to classes. It was difficult to believe summer was over, leaving me in the same condition I had been in in June. I couldn't help but compare my image in the mirror with the one I had seen a year earlier.

Today I saw a fragile woman with tired eyes, hair standing up in thin wisps. She was a frail, sick bird not long for this world, or definitely working a limited engagement. Charlie, holding me in his arms in the kitchen, said, "My little Jill, I can feel your heart beating." In cutting off my breast, my heart had been exposed emotionally and physically. I had lost my insulation, my padding, both literally and figuratively. I was so low I felt that if I stopped fighting and closed my eyes, I would just drift away and die.

I told Sue how low I felt and about the piercing pain I was experiencing in my right knee, which I attributed to the Los Angeles sauna condition. The humidity was cruel. I complained that everyone else was living my life while I watched. My friends were riding my horses. They were swimming in the ocean for me and sometimes even eating and drinking for me. I didn't like it. We discussed whether I was ready to give up riding and running my horse business. Was I finished with that phase of my life? For some time now the signs had been pointing in that direction. My arthritis was worse. For the past two years riding had become increasingly difficult, but I found it hard to let it go. I was scared of giving in, giving up. She said maybe closing the chapter on one thing opened up the next chapter, but I didn't find much comfort in that. I rested in relaxed conversation for an hour, then drove home.

It was becoming increasingly difficult to handle my illness gracefully. I had been suffering from diarrhea for three days, I had a sore bottom and the lack of hair on my head made me look like a newly hatched bird. That afternoon I asked my daughter, "I bet you can't remember the last time I was well and fun, can you?"

Zuleika gave me her straight-from-the-shoulder, level-eyed look. "Yes, I can, Mom. When you had Limo and I had Cadok."

They were two horses we owned. I was grateful Zuleika remembered me whole. I had almost forgotten. Thank God she hadn't.

It took four days to recover from chemotherapy number four. By Thursday my system seemed to kick over. I was able to regroup and pick up the fight once more.

Alan came to trim what was left of my hair. It didn't feel like hair anymore, more like clammy cotton. I made him cut it extremely short. Alan, in a silly mood, said I looked like Joan of Arc. True, my head was almost shaved. Alan struck a pose. "That's what you get for sleeping with enemy soldiers."

He had cut my hair in the downstairs powder room. Now I dashed upstairs to my bathroom to shower off the bits of hair. On my way up the stairs, I passed Charlie on his way down. He stopped at the sight of me. We stood on the stairs eye-to-eye. He was stunned. My head showed all the bald spots, exposed, sunburned pink and gleaming; I was not at all the English rose he'd fallen in love with so many years before. We continued to stare, and as I looked into his eyes I saw so many thoughts and emotions flood across his face that I felt a short, stabbing pang of pain for him and the past. Then, just as swiftly, I moved through it.

"I don't care, darling, I really don't. It feels better this way."

Charlie, wordlessly, passed me and walked out onto the balcony to sit, staring out at the ocean. I didn't care. It *did* feel better. I found it hard to believe that only five months before, I had been sitting in a sumptuous suite in the George V Hotel in Paris preparing to attend the César Awards, the French Oscars.

With diamonds twinkling in my ears and at my throat, sipping champagne and chatting with Charlie, I wore a beautiful white silk silver-beaded gown from Chanel's new collection. It was a very cold February, and over my gown I was swaddled in a floor-length white fox fur. Charlie, handsome in his tuxedo, told me how proud he was of the way I looked this evening. As we walked through the elegant lobby, I could feel his pride when people turned to watch our progress to the waiting limousine at the curb.

As we drove through the hordes of excited spectators on the way to the theater, I heard the name Bronson, Bronson, Bronson repeated as admiring faces peered into the back of our elegant transport. As I was handed out of the car, I caught the eyes of many women enviously admiring my clothes, my jewels, my husband, my looks. How many of them would have traded places with me had they known that a tumor within me maliciously grew larger every day?

I indulged myself one moment longer in that lovely time when I hadn't known what was in store for me. Then I slapped on a hat and went out on the veranda to where Charlie was sitting. I stood behind him and put my arms around him.

"Don't feel bad, Charlie. My hair will grow back. Alan saw some regrowth coming in already."

I kissed the side of his neck as he patted my hand. I said, "I'm going to the barn. I'll see you later. I love you."

My lovely, older horse, named Cadok, was once a very fancy, winning show hunter, but he had been badly injured while being vanned to a show. Now he was recuperating, his show career over. He was still my favorite and the one I liked to ride best. I regularly took him to Vermont for R and R after the stresses of the show circuit. This day I watched Cadok in the turnout ring, walking lazily around sniffing the ground. He came over to where I stood by the rail and looked at me inquiringly.

"Hi, Cadok, old boy. You and I have been having a rough time, but we're going to make it. We'll be just fine, you'll see." He stood beside me, listening, occasionally sniffing my hair. I stroked his neck and felt peaceful.

I had been keeping my mother's fears at bay, telephoning her often to say I was fine, but she had reached a point, as she put it, where she had to see for herself. So my seventy-nine-year-old mother put my father in a rest home for two weeks, then flew alone to Los Angeles. Packing a silver tea set, two crystal vases, some English chocolates and an old scrapbook of photographs, she bravely climbed aboard a plane to travel alone for the first time in her life.

Paul met his grandmother at the airport and drove her to the beach house. She was obviously exhausted, having been awake nearly twenty-four hours. But she was alert, full of snappy, tart comments, relieved to see me looking "much better than I had imagined."

Together, we unpacked her suitcase, hanging up her few articles of clothing. Her bag was mostly filled by the tea set and crystal.

"Oh, Mummy, what are these for?"

"Well, I have no use for such things anymore." Then she said sweetly, "I wanted to bring you something."

"Well, I love them. Thank you, Mummy."

I gave her a gentle hug and a kiss. Her fatigue was showing now and her small body felt frail as I held her. Her skin was soft. As I held her hands, I marveled at how fragile they were. She is a lovely old lady with very white, soft, fluffy hair cut short to frame her face. Her eyes are bright blue and knowing. Looking at her today, so tired, but so valiant and determined,

I thought she was the most lovely old lady I had ever seen.

It gave me a warm, cozy feeling that night, knowing my mother was under the same roof. My mother had come to me. It was as if the act itself had the power to heal.

As the days passed by lazily and happily, I told her all about Sue Colin and holistic medicine and Bernard Dowson and homeopathic healing. I gave her a crystal and led her through some meditation. I sat with her, Zuleika and Katrina, and we meditated together.

One day, I showed her my scar. She looked at it carefully and said, "It's what I imagined; it's not so bad, Jilly. Though I would willingly have had it instead of you. I would have given both of my old breasts to have you keep your young one."

She was as encouraging and determined for me as she had been years ago when, hand in hand, we entered the magic world of ballet, lights and music. From my seat on the veranda, I watched her standing on the beach, a small, upright figure. The distance between us melted away the years, making invisible the many wrinkles in the sunburned skin, so that only her resoluteness and vitality showed. I felt her strength of spirit as she stood, shoulders back, head up, her strong profile tipped upward toward the sun, legs braced apart, balancing firmly on her deformed feet, which were crippled and sore with arthritis and bunions. At this moment, my mother looked to be much younger. I felt my heart fill with pride and my eyes, with tears.

She stayed the two weeks; then satisfied with my condition, she began to worry about my father. Saying, "My life is in England. That's where I belong," she thanked Charlie for having her and for being so good to her daughter. Then home she went with a hug, a kiss and an "I love you, Jilly." Leaving behind one tea set, two vases, some chocolate and more than a little bit of her strength and determination with her daughter, my mother returned to my father.

16

I PICKED UP MY ROUTINE AGAIN. Meditate in the morning upon rising, see the girls off to school, drive to see Sue Colin or Bernard Dowson, come home, have lunch, meditate again. The afternoons were spent on the beach or at the stables with Zuleika. In the evenings I helped the girls with their homework, had dinner and meditated again before bed.

I was nervous about Bernard Dowson's treatments. After all, going to him twice a week, lying on his electromagnetic wave table, drinking electrically charged water four times a day, by most people's standards was unorthodox. What if the table stimulated cancer cells and made them grow faster? Bernard said cancer couldn't survive those vibrations. I didn't understand the table, yet I had no choice but to trust him if I were to continue to see him. The saliva tests and electrical acupuncture clamps on my ear combined with the hair snip enabled him to determine how I was progressing. He told me I was doing well, that my health and energy had improved significantly and that I would be fine.

Bernard ran a number of allergy tests on me and gave me a list of foods to which I was allergic. These I began to exclude from my diet. He also practiced what he called broadcasting. He used my hair snip, saying, "Your body creates a specific order, a specific pattern. Just like snowflakes, there are no two exactly the same. There are no two humans, no two genetic patterns, no two pieces of hair that are exactly the same. Every part of your body has a code. It's like having a safe with a thousand-digit combination; your body and your hair have exactly the same unique code. There's a resonance. When you change, your hair changes, too, for a while, until it loses the pattern and fades away."

I interjected, "That sounds like what witch doctors do."

He replied, "Exactly. In voodoo, hair and nails are taken from a person. You can be anywhere in the world and that's enough. The kahunas of Hawaii do all their healing through the mechanism — at a distance."

It was weird all right, but I continued to see him. All the territory I traveled was new and uncharted, and I had to go with my inner feelings. At least Michael Van Scoy Mosher, who had said he had nothing against homeopathy except that there was no way to know if it worked, had an open mind. I didn't dare tell Ray Weston all the stuff Bernard did. I could imagine how loudly he would say, "Quack, quack, quack!"

I did some research at UCLA's Bio Lab Medical Library and learned, interestingly enough, that a table very much like Bernard's was being used in Sweden. And in Russia they were treating cancer with electromagnetic waves. In the *Smithsonian,* there was an article by Jack Fincher entitled "New Machines May Soon Replace the Doctor's Black Bag." From this and others, I read that the body has its own magnetic fields. The introduction of electromagnetics stimulates injuries, promoting faster healing.

Every time I read something about cancer, I felt the familiar stirrings of fear. The message I was getting from everyone — from doctors, scientists, homeopaths, holistic healers, psychiatrists and oncologists — was that there *is* such a thing as a cancer personality. If patients weren't prepared to make changes in their lives, their chances of recovery would be considerably reduced. Bernard thought I had become ill because my mind, not my body, broke down.

Every day I felt happier, better than I had for a long, long time. Occasional reminders of the monster were not so bad — not even so unwelcome. They kept me in touch with the reality of my situation.

Getting well was like any other job. It had highs and lows. The important thing was to keep up the work. In the mornings I said to myself, "Well, come on, get up and get on with your job." During setbacks, I told myself, "Keep chipping away, do the cancer meditation." I did the "white cells fighting the cancer cells" imagery and tried to be true to myself to reduce stress. I began delegating responsibilities. My secretary, Sue Overholt, took over Zuleika Farm West. Charlie began driving Zuleika to and from her riding lessons. I taught Katrina to be more independent, telling her that when she did things for herself she became stronger, but when I did things for her it robbed me of precious energy I needed to heal myself. I became more truthful with myself about what I really wanted to do with my time. I stopped doing things because I thought I should. My personal goals were to become completely well, to write a book I hoped would be a companion for others going through similar trials and if I could, to be less hard on myself, to accept and like myself just as I was. I would work on filling my life with good quality time.

Dr. O. Carl Simonton asked his patients to list eight stresses they had suffered during the eighteen months prior to their cancer. According to Dr. Simonton, there was no way I could have avoided becoming seriously ill. I had touched all the bases.

I believe I could have withstood one or perhaps two of the traumas during that period. I had in the past. But somehow this combination was too much. Toward the end of the eighteen months prior to becoming ill, I definitely was stressed out. But I could not halt the pattern. I had not taken time to replenish my energies. I had become deeply depressed. My white blood cells had stopped doing their job. When I stopped fighting, they stopped fighting. White blood cells kill off millions of cancer cells over and over again during a lifetime. There are always cancer cells in our bodies. The only time they grow and multiply is when our white blood cells allow it. I'll never know at what point I was drained. I don't know what I could have done to insulate myself against the shocks and bereavements of that difficult period. Would meditation have helped? Could I have tapped into the universe and taken of its energy to help heal myself as I was trying to do now? If I'd been going to Bernard Dowson, would his electromagnetic wave table have kept me healthy? Could I have withstood my troubles without becoming ill? Without becoming a cancer victim?

I wanted to live a long time. Sometimes the thought obsessed me. I felt as if I were only just learning how to live, and I saw the possibility of life becoming even more fulfilling. I was not about to let it be taken away from me.

Charlie had mellowed. He was softer somehow, more gentle with me. We still had occasional spats, but they were rare. I was completely uninhibited with my husband. He accepted me and the surgery. It seemed to make no difference to him. It certainly hadn't affected our sex life, and it speaks for the man, as well as our relationship, that it never occurred to me that it would. Indeed, Charlie and I made love with the same tenderness and passion that we had for the last twenty years.

After a couple of months, I also walked around naked as I always had in front of him. He would kiss the scar and tell me, "I don't feel any differently about you. It doesn't make any difference to me."

And I believed him. Yes, if the only reason I had to live was my husband, I wanted to live a long, long time. The thought that something could take away my life and happiness scared me. I didn't want to die.

It is true, though, that cancer has tremendously rewarding sides. I became closer to my family and friends; the ones I now knew as friends were not a large army, but a few. The ones who stayed close were those who genuinely felt about me the way I felt toward them. Who and what I am as a woman does not depend on my physical appearance. Nor does it matter to them if I am sick or well. I am still Jill. Deep inside I knew I hadn't changed. I didn't need two breasts to be a woman. I knew I was a woman; the things that made me *me* were untouched. I was the same. In fact, I was opening doors, making discoveries about myself that would have taken years without the illness. It would be unfair to make all these discoveries only to lose them.

The real estate broker called about the House That Jack Built. "I think they're going to take your bid, Jill. They've bid on a house they want to buy. We have to wait a few days to see if it is accepted. If so, then they'll take your bid."

I couldn't wait to tell Charlie. Each time I saw the House That Jack Built I became full of happy plans, wondering which of my favorite pieces of antique furniture would fit. My house. It stood for a great deal. I ached for the challenge of restoring it to its former glory. I wanted to start work on it. If I had my house, I couldn't die. I needed at least twenty years in it!

My optimism about the house was only slightly dimmed by the reality that chemotherapy number five was only a week away. As yet, I didn't feel the gripping panic. I hoped I wouldn't. Maybe this time I could simply go along, receive the injection, go home, be a little sick and feel fine the next day. I tried to do as much riding as possible before my treatment. Now, as early as ten weeks after surgery, I was riding Cadok for an hour almost every morning. I also rode Robbie, a beautiful gray thoroughbred — two horses a day. I was proud of myself.

Zuleika Farm West had ten horses. With my illness, I called in all my horsemen friends to help. Sue Overholt, my secretary, is a horsewoman. In the mornings she helped turn out and exercise all the horses. A real estate broker friend, Mark Farndale, an excellent horseman, worked the horses in the evenings. Another friend, Kathy Kuzner, twice an Olympian who once held the equestrian high-jump record, gave Zuleika lessons. Under Kathy's tutelage, Zuleika's riding improved substantially.

I was growing stronger, although realistically I had to

admit it would be a long time before I could ride four horses a day as I had in the past. With help from my friends, Zuleika Farm West flourished. Alan would run here and there, working like a demon, while insulting me with gusto. "You're an eccentric, friggin' old Empress," he'd yell as I asked him to do yet another chore.

I was anything but an empress when I visited Michael. My blood count was acceptably low, as he had planned it.

He said, "We try to keep the blood cells down just a little. That way we know the chemo is getting to you."

I must have gained confidence, because I slipped chocolate into my diet one night. Then I began eating wheat. I continued to tempt fate, giving my willpower a vacation. I was feeling good and nothing happened for a few days. Then I noticed that at four every afternoon I was hit by gripping headaches. I put them down to the heat. But after three days of terrible discomfort I decided Bernard Dowson's assessment was correct. Since the headaches were new, I concluded that I really was allergic to caffeine, chocolate and wheat. I stopped eating them, and the headaches disappeared.

17

ONE MORNING AFTER MY daily walk with my big German shepherd, Cassie, I joined Charlie for breakfast on the veranda. I gave him a kiss, then, comfortably ensconced in my favorite couch, I slowly ate breakfast while thumbing through some fashion magazines. I liked the look of a black velvet dress, so I tore out the page to remind me to track it down. I already imagined myself in the gown, elegant and soignée. I never gave my scalped head a thought.

I sat happily dreaming about clothes and glamorous evenings when I became aware of a terrifyingly familiar feeling in my remaining breast. Oh, God, it was burning and tingling. I remembered the sensation. It struck before I had the biopsy in my right breast.

And now I felt the burning and tingling again. I tentatively felt around and discovered a lump. Goddammit, a goddamn, fucking lump. Fear surged through me. A lump! A lump! Oh, God, I can't go through it again. I knew my surgeon was out of town for three weeks. Should I go to his office and see his associate? I spoke to Charlie.

"Charlie, I have another lump."

He looked at me. "When do you see Dr. Karlan?"

"He's away for two more weeks."

"I know this is bad stuff, Jill. Bad stuff has been happening to you, really bad stuff, but you are on chemotherapy. Try not to worry; maybe it's just a gland."

I kissed him good-bye and left for my appointment with Bernard Dowson. Alan, who noticed I was down, packed me into the car.

"What's up, girl?"

"I've got another lump in my breast."

He looked stricken. "We've got to sit down and talk to Dowson. Let's go."

I sat beside Alan, fear rippling through me. I couldn't push away the thought that somehow I was going to lose my left breast, too.

I lay on Bernard's electromagnetic table trying to meditate and visualize my white blood cells attacking and killing any cancer they found, but I was too anxious. The table made me feel feverish. I was frightened. I wanted to jump off and get out of there. But I waited for the thirty minutes to pass and then went downstairs to the reception area, where Alan waited, to talk to Bernard. Alan did the talking.

"Bernard, Jill has another lump and we want to know how she is doing. We're not playing patty-cake here, Bernard. This is serious. What's going on?"

I joined in. "I'm afraid of the table. Maybe it is stimulating my cancer cells."

Bernard shook his head. "No it isn't," he said definitely. He told me once again how electromagnetic waves were being used in Russia and Sweden to treat cancer. It was early, but it was a breakthrough. I was one of the first to be treated with this method. I really didn't understand, but once again Bernard gave me confidence in what he was doing. I asked him to find out what was happening by checking my hair. He said I was doing very well — the cancer was sixty percent gone the last time he'd tested my hair — and that I was getting better and better. He was sure I had nothing to worry about and asked me to call him in an hour. Somehow this reassured me. Bernard's supplementary care was a nice addition to my AMA treatment. It was so strange; having this illness was either mind-expanding or else I was going crazy. Imagine believing all this!

Alan gave me a big, comforting hug. I felt so vulnerable. But I was also concerned for Alan. He took it all so intensely. He cared so much. We went to the Good Earth restaurant for lunch. Eating cheered us up. We took the leftovers to the car for Cassie, and drove home.

When we arrived, Alan immediately telephoned Bernard, who talked to both of us. Bernard thought a lymph gland was responsible for the lump. I probably had a virus. As far as he could determine, the cancer was gone.

What Charlie made of all this, I don't know. He knew that whatever he said about homeopathy might be negative and I wouldn't want to hear it. I was following my own intuition. If someone as important to me as Charlie had come down strongly against the whole thing, it would genuinely have upset me, so he kept his peace and watched.

Later, Charlie and I took a long walk on the beach, discussing the house we hoped to buy. The owners had turned down our bid again. We were disappointed. The owners, in our opinion, had greatly overpriced the house in the first place. We thought it was worth only two-thirds of what they were asking, and it needed much work. In spite of this, we again decided to up our offer, really for the beach location. I have to admit my emotions were clouding my business judgment, and I was dragging Charlie along with me, reluctantly, I might add.

The Bel Air house had definitely been a fixer-upper, too, when we bought it. In the early years we couldn't afford to do much to it, so we painted the walls off-white, replaced the carpets and curtains and threw afghans over the multicolored couches and chairs. Our walls were decorated with paintings that we had done, including a large, masterful work by Charlie of a coal miner sitting in a round wooden tub, fatigued and grimy from the day's work, with his wife washing his back. Ignoring the awesomeness of the task, I bullied the house into shape with the many odds and ends we brought from our other houses. At night, in the glow of the many candles used to disguise the decorating inadequacies, the old house took on what I liked to think was an elegantly shabby appearance.

But as our prosperity grew, we added antique furnishings and objects of art from all over the world: country French end tables, tapestries from Turkey, an enormous grandfather clock from Germany (wound religiously by Charlie), paintings and bronzes from Paris and London. I never did use a decorator, but rather tried to re-create the warm atmosphere of an English country house. What a tremendous job it had been, but after seventeen years it was comfortable and quite beautiful. An enormous responsibility, it had everything we wanted and then some — the "then some" was what I wanted to dispose of. I now needed my energy for other things. I resented using my power reserve on inanimate objects, possessions.

The House That Jack Built, smaller, simpler, was perfect for us. There were two run-down outbuildings; one to become an office, the other I envisioned as Charlie's exercise room.

I was determined the House That Jack Built would be completely overhauled, its face lifted and painted, before we moved in. It didn't occur to me for a moment we wouldn't get the house, even though the owner was definitely negative about negotiating. I knew the house was for me. Charlie was concerned I'd be disappointed. "Don't get your heart set on this house, Jill. We may not be able to get it."

It was September, and the next day, some four months after my surgery, Charlie's older sister Antorchia died. She had had a very sad life. As a child Antorchia contracted scarlet fever. The illness left her deaf. She never learned to speak, and spent her life in silence, unable to communicate except by a very old sign language, a method no longer in use and which few people understood. Saddened, Charlie said Antorchia needed his support at the funeral. He was concerned there would be few mourners, so my husband flew to Pennsylvania.

During the two days he was away, the real estate lady called and told me the owners had accepted our new bid. I waited until Charlie came home to tell him the news. Charlie arrived proud and pleased at how many people had attended Antorchia's funeral. One old man of eighty old him, "Your sister was a real beauty when she was a young girl. When I read she had died, I just had to come to her funeral. She was a real beauty."

The trip to Pennsylvania, among relatives and old friends, obviously had moved Charlie, so I waited before telling him our special news. When I did, he was sitting on the veranda looking out at the ocean. I came and knelt beside him.

"I've got some wonderful news, darling."

"What is it?"

"What do you think? Something very important to both of us."

He looked long and hard at me. He didn't say anything.

"It's the house. We can have the house. They accepted our bid."

Charlie ran his hands through his hair, more in horror than in joy.

"You're kidding?"

"No, I'm not kidding. It's going to be *our* house."

Charlie was stunned. He loved our Bel Air home. He was sad knowing it would mean selling the house. Moving to the beach had become a reality.

In the days that followed, Charlie caught the excitement. We planned how we would design his exercise room and the office. I was happy as I watched my excitement affect him. Zuleika and Katrina were thrilled. The older children were unhappy. They had lived many happy years in the Bel Air home. It held special memories for them.

I suggested before we left the house we have one last family dinner in the dining room.

"That's a terrible idea," Paul said. "Can you imagine us sitting there, saying this is the last time. Don't do that, whatever you do."

I promised I wouldn't. "But don't worry, boys. It's going to be at least two years before the house is sold." That seemed to mollify them. At least they would have time to adjust.

I knew when the time came, I would be sad at leaving the

house. I, too, had time to adjust. But whenever I spoke of the future, I got a strange feeling. Perhaps it was when I spoke of time in years. It's true, nobody knows the future. People become ill and die every day. But when you've had cancer, you see things a little differently . . . and you hope. You hope.

18

EVEN AS THE FIFTH chemotherapy treatment loomed ahead I was enjoying the golden days, one tranquility that Malibu had to offer.

The Saturday before my fifth treatment, Zuleika, Charlie and I were going to attend the United States Equestrian Team Finals at Griffith Park. As usual for my forays into the other world, I tried to look as well as possible. I carefully made up my eyes, putting blue kohl on the inside of my lids and lots of mascara on my lashes. I covered my head with a bright red Garboesque straw hat. I wore a red linen dress and sandals. I looked at myself in the mirror. As long as no one knocked my hat off, I'd probably still knock 'em dead in the aisles, as they say.

The possibility of my hat falling off was a real fear. I had lunched recently with an agent. I had dressed carefully in a safari-type outfit with a dashing hat. Lunch went smoothly. I thought I had made a good impression. As I walked elegantly out, I paused on the street to say good-bye. The restaurant was on a corner. A sudden gust of wind came whipping around and blew off my hat. I was exposed. The hat rolled gaily down the street while I watched helplessly. Everyone stared at my head. I had to laugh. What a waste of effort and all the careful primping. Oh, well, what the hell. I said good-bye as if nothing were amiss, pretending I simply sported the latest in punk rock haircuts and watched the doorman gallantly chase down my hat.

I hoped nothing of the sort would happen at the horse show. The "other world" was populated by people not connected with my everyday life, a world I had carelessly taken for granted before I knew I had cancer. All the souls close to me were accustomed to my hair and my occasional down days. I had asked Zuleika one day, "Were you worried, darling, when you knew I had cancer?"

"No. I knew you'd be all right."

"How did you know?"

"Because I can see you, and you are."

I loved that.

I enjoyed seeing friends at the championships, and watching the competitors ride so well. It became cold during the day and my elegance came undone. Charlie, concerned I would catch cold, bought me a gray cotton sweat suit, insisting I wear it. The pants went on underneath my stylish red linen dress and the top went over it, leaving me clad in the sweat suit, red hat, diamond earrings and high-heeled sandals. The ensemble kept me warm, but was hardly the image I had set out to project. However, I soon forgot my appearance in the enjoyment of the day. Everyone related to me openly and freely. They seemed delighted to see me so cheerful. I suppose people expected me to look much worse; instead, with my makeup and bright red hat covering my bald patches, I looked quite well. So things weren't so bad after all.

Zuleika wasn't competing in the event, nevertheless she enjoyed cheering on her friends. We sat at one of the many round tables, eating hot dogs while she chatted excitedly, watching the competitors.

In spite of the cold, we stayed until the completion of the show, then drove home. Cassie, who had been left behind, greeted me enthusiastically, with many squeals, yelps and much jumping about.

That night after kissing Zuleika good night, I put on pajamas and sat cross-legged on the bedroom floor. With a crystal in each hand I tried to meditate. Instead, I found myself thinking of my daughter. With a sudden urgency, the fear I had been repressing surfaced: what if cancer struck Zuleika and I wasn't there to help her? I had read repeatedly how cancer ran in families and was considered hereditary. I would give anything, even my life, to be sure she would never have to go through that. But if, God forbid, in the future it did happen — rage filled me with hatred at the thought — I determined to be a good example, to arm her with positive memories of how her mother had handled the challenge.

Once again I cursed the malignancy and vowed to get it all back — looks, health, everything. This time for my daughter and her future.

Oh, Zuleika, that special, beloved child. I had brought to the bedroom at the beach house my favorite photograph of Zuleika and me, taken when she was about four. She was sitting on my lap, facing me, her head tipped to one side and pressed against my breast. Oh, she loved her Mama, as she called me then. Taped to the right-hand corner of the frame was a little gold whistle. It reminded me of the day the photograph was taken.

Zuleika had accompanied me to a rehearsal for the 1976 Hollywood Foreign Press Association's Golden Globe Awards. I was to peform the title song from the movie *From Noon Till Three,* which had been nominated for the best song award. The film remains Charlie's and my favorite of the dozen or so movies in which we worked together. The show was being televised the following day. Charlie was out of town finishing work in a new film. Zuleika was my little buddy and biggest fan. She loved the song and thought her mother had the most beautiful voice in the world.

I would sing the lyrics to her every night before she went to sleep. She remembered every line and sang along with me, lying on her back with her eyes on mine, her hand twisting a lock of my hair as we crooned together. As I looked at the photograph I found myself singing the song quietly:

> *Some have a lifetime, some just a day.*
> *Love isn't something you measure that way.*

Nothing's ever for ever.
Forever's a lie.
All we have is between Hello and Good-bye.

Many celebrities were assembled for the awards show, among them Barbra Streisand and Raquel Welch. Melissa Manchester was friendly at the rehearsals, as was Paul Williams, who helped me rehearse with the piano.

Zuleika had been so excited about my being on TV singing her favorite song; she fussed around the Beverly Wilshire Hotel suite that I used as a dressing room. As I changed into my beautiful black velvet gown, which Bob Mackie had made for me, Zuleika and her nanny visited the hotel gift shop and bought me the gold whistle charm for luck. She pinned the whistle to the lining of the dress. It was a simple gown, strapless, low-cut with a deep V neck. Zuleika said I looked beautiful. Now that dress was hanging in the large cedar closet that houses most of my formal gowns. I never wore it again, and now because of the deep décolletage I knew I never would.

Now Zuleika was a teenager and Katrina had grown from a skinny little girl into a lovely sixteen-year-old. I talked to a friend in advertising about the girls' prospects as models. Susie Dotan said, "Sure, let's take some test shots this weekend. *Teen* magazine is looking for young girls. I think Zuleika would be perfect for a certain ad I have in mind."

I asked my trusty friend Alan to do their makeup and hair. I found myself in the role of stage mother, running around getting cups of tea, finding hair dryers, searching my wardrobe for suitable outfits for the girls. Zuleika, made up, her hair blown dry, was gorgeous. Susie and the photographer set up upstairs on the veranda, where Zuleika would have a background of turquoise ocean to accentuate her blond hair and turquoise eyes. I hovered, watching, then went downstairs to see how Katrina was coming along. She was made up in a more grown-up fashion. Alan had transformed the sixteen-year-old girl into a beautiful, sultry brunette who looked eighteen.

Alan chattered happily. He told the girls, "I remember when I did this for your mother in the old days." I felt as if I were a hundred, definitely an out-of-date model.

Alan caught my eye. "Lovely young things. Come on, you old bag, come and stand next to me." He put his arm around me affectionately. We stood together watching "the babies," as he called them. Zuleika, shy and tentative; Katrina, a bit more confident, more sure of her womanhood.

Poor Charlie had been kicked off his favorite afternoon spot on the veranda to make way for the photographers. He saw Zuleika walk down the stairs in full makeup. He looked shocked.

"I didn't look too closely, Jill, because I might not have approved of something and I didn't want to say anything."

"Don't worry, darling, she looks beautiful. The light washes out most of the makeup anyway. You know that."

Charlie looked uncertain. "Mmm, hmm," he said and went off to find another retreat where he could stay out of the way and read.

It made for a pleasant afternoon. Zuleika was particularly delighted, as it postponed her dreaded homework, for a time anyway. I was getting a taste of things to come. My two young ladies. This was the year Katrina would learn to drive and Charlie was going to buy her a car. Oh boy! I'd seen five teenagers grow up, drive cars and eventually arrive safely at their twenties. I knew what was coming. I mentally braced myself for the long nights of sitting, waiting for Katrina to drive home. Charlie and I customarily sat in the study waiting for one of our new drivers to arrive home. At every screech and slamming of brakes on Sunset Boulevard, Charlie would spring to his feet, saying, "Oh, God, I hope that's not Valentine or Jason." They all survived and made it out of their teens safely. I knew Katrina would, too.

I wanted to live for the next five years cancer-free. I knew that would be a good sign and I would be considered in remission. Yet I didn't want to wish my life away so quickly. The next five years were going to be important. Bernard advised, "You should have more quality time, Jill. Try to fill your life with things you enjoy." Today, photographing the girls, was one of those days. I had enjoyed myself. I could still live, love and laugh with one breast. There were moments of loneliness and fear when the monster visited me. But those times seemed to heighten my pleasures. Simple things were so lovely — the sun on my face, my love for my husband, the feel of my daughters as I held them in my arms, the love that flooded my senses when I embraced my sons, the exhilaration when I watched my dogs running full of energy across an open space. I knew I wouldn't change anything. I wouldn't give my cancer back. Time is running out for all of us. We know as we are born the clock starts ticking. Sometimes I'd thought that quality, not quantity, was important. But now I wanted it all. All of it for as long as I could. The rewards were so great, the battle so worth fighting.

There was one more week to go before chemo five. I tried to stay in the moment and not think about chemotherapy. In the coming week Dr. Karlan would examine the lump in my left breast. There was no sense of foreboding because I did not feel the presence of cancer now. The burning and tingling sensation had diminished. Maybe all would be well.

19

I TAPED A MEDITATION from Dr. Simonton's book, *Getting Well Again,* with the sound of the Malibu surf pounding in the background. The intimate sound of my voice reached directly into my subconscious. Soothingly it suggested that I would get well. Each night I listened to myself recite:

2. Become aware of your breathing.

3. Take in a few deep breaths and, as you let out each breath, mentally say the word, "relax."

4. Concentrate on your face and feel any tension in the muscles of your face and around your eyes. Make a mental picture of this tension — it might be a rope tied in a knot or a clenched fist — and then mentally picture it relaxing and becoming comfortable, like a limp rubber band.

5. Experience the muscles of your face and eyes becoming relaxed. As they relax, feel a wave of relaxation spreading through your body.

6. Tense the muscles of your face and around your eyes, squeezing tightly, then relax them and feel the relaxation spreading through your body.

7. Move slowly down your body — jaw, neck, shoulders, back, upper and lower arms, hands, chest, abdomen, thighs, calves, ankles, feet — until every part of your body is more relaxed. For each part of the body, mentally picture the tension, then picture the tension melting away, allowing relaxation.

8. Now picture yourself in pleasant, natural surroundings — wherever feels comfortable for you. Mentally fill in the details of color, sound, texture.

9. Continue to picture yourself in a very relaxed state in this natural place for two or three minutes.

10. Then mentally picture the cancer in either realistic or symbolic terms. Think of the cancer as consisting of very weak, confused cells. Remember that our bodies destroy cancerous cells thousands of times during a normal lifetime. As you picture your cancer, realize that your recovery requires that your body's own defenses return to a natural, healthy state.

11. . . . If you are receiving chemotherapy, picture that drug coming into your body and entering the bloodstream. Picture the drug acting like a poison. The normal cells are intelligent and strong and don't take up the poison so readily. But the cancer cell is a weak cell, so it takes very little to kill it. It absorbs the poison, dies, and is flushed out of your body.

12. Picture your body's own white blood cells coming into the area where the cancer is, recognizing the abnormal cells, and destroying them. There is a vast army of white blood cells. They are very strong and aggressive. They are also very smart. There is no contest between them and the cancer cells: they will win the battle.

13. Picture the cancer shrinking. See the dead cells being carried away by the white blood cells and being flushed from your body through the liver and kidneys and eliminated in the urine and stool. This is your expectancy of what you want to happen. Continue to see the cancer shrinking, until it is all gone. See yourself having more energy and a better appetite and being able to feel comfortable and loved in your family as the cancer shrinks and finally disappears.

14. If you are experiencing pain anywhere in your body, picture the army of white blood cells flowing into that area and soothing the pain. Whatever the problem, give your body the command to heal itself. Visualize your body becoming well.

15. Imagine yourself well, free of disease, full of energy.

16. Picture yourself reaching your goals in life. See your purpose in life being fulfilled, the members of your family doing well, your relationships with people around you becoming more meaningful. Remember that having strong reasons for being well will help you to get well, so use this time to focus clearly on your priorities in life.

17. Now give yourself a mental pat on the back for participating in your recovery. See yourself doing this mental imagery exercise three times a day, staying awake and alert as you do it.

18. Then let the muscles in your eyelids lighten up, become ready to open your eyes, and become aware of the room.

19. Now let your eyes open, and you are ready to resume your usual activities.

As had Bernard Dowson, Dr. Simonton told me to fill my days with quality time, avoiding stress. At first it was difficult to recognize the difference between what I thought I should do and what I needed to do. Gradually, I was getting better at it.

What surprised me was nobody else seemed to notice the difference. I had assumed all the chores and obligations over the years because I had convinced myself I was the only one who could handle them. Now they were being discharged by friends and members of my family. I wasn't missed. I must have been driving myself, or was it that cancer gave me an excuse, putting me in a position to be myself, to do what I wanted and to avoid the unnecessary? No one else seemed overburdened or overstressed by my withdrawal from the frantic field of action. It was something to think about.

Women my age were reared to live their lives for their husbands and families. This may be wondrous and noble, but not healthful. Perhaps that overly supportive role contributes to breast cancer.

I remembered my days as a young actress in England working in live TV. There was a countdown: ten, nine, eight, seven, six, five, four, three, two, one — and then someone would tap me on the shoulder (the stage manager usually) and back out of the picture. I'd be on my own without a net for as long as the play lasted. I felt I was living that way now — to the hilt, without a safety net.

Sue Colin had been away for ten days and today, finally, I was to see her. I had slept badly, too tired to meditate. I put a banana, some fruit juice and protein powder in a blender and drank my breakfast, then drove to her office. She could see I was tired and dispirited. I told her how tired I was, and I also told Sue about my wonderful week, when I had been full of energy. I confessed I'd gone off my diet, eating cookies.

"Ah ha," she said, "that would make you tired. You know what sugar does to you." I nodded, feeling guilty. Could all this fatigue be as simple as that?

Sue and I discussed my forthcoming meeting with Mitchell Karlan to examine the lump in my left breast, and how angry I was when I'd discovered it. When the hour was up, my fatigue had miraculously disappeared. I left Sue's office feeling more at ease with myself, and carrying a poster she had loaned me "to live with for a while." It depicted a setting sun with a tree in the foreground. Written in the corner was the inscription *The Five Freedoms:*

- To see and hear what is here instead of what should be, was, or will be.
- To say what one feels and thinks instead of what one should do.
- To feel what one feels instead of what one ought.
- To ask for what one wants instead of always waiting for permission.
- To take risks on one's own behalf instead of choosing to be only secure and not rocking the boat.

It was written by Virginia Sateer, a therapist who, Sue said, had been a cancer victim. The five admonitions seemed very personal to someone dealing with cancer. Maybe I would incorporate them into my own meditation tapes.

In my car I turned the radio to rock and roll, which energized me. I like Mick Jagger particularly. His earthy, gritty, raucous sound always seemed to pick me up. I wished I could sing and move like Tina Turner. Yes, that's the kind of energy I could use right now — a touch of old "Proud Mary."

When I arrived home, I rode Cadok while Pesty, my young, talented equestrian friend, exercised a couple of other horses for me. I enjoyed a pleasant afternoon, but as the day wore on a throbbing headache hit me. By six o'clock my head was in a vise of pain. I ate dinner hoping food would shift it. But it didn't. Charlie sat me in front of him on his chair and massaged the back of my neck and temples. This helped — at least his closeness relaxed me a little.

"I think it's tension, baby. I think you're worried about tomorrow and seeing Dr. Karlan."

Two Ascriptin A/D and a five-milligram Valium helped. I hated to think that despite my efforts to try to live in the moment, deep down inside, nagging away, was a fear causing my terrible headache. If worry caused the headache, what else might it cause? That question produced more tension, increasing the pain. As the evening wore on, Charlie continued massaging my neck and shoulders, which helped relieve the tension. It also made me grateful for the sympathy.

By bedtime, I admitted to myself the pain was probably a product of anxiety about Mitchell's examination the following day, but I was disappointed because I believed I had worry under control. Maybe it was fatigue. Maybe I'd done too much the previous week. Maybe I was getting a cold. These thoughts produced more worry. What if I had a cold Monday when I was due for chemotherapy? I must control the worry and force my mind to relax. At eleven o'clock, I said to Charlie, "You watch the news. I'm going to meditate. It should help get rid of the headache."

"I'll see you up there," he replied.

I mounted the stairs, sat on the bed with the tape player, selected a large amethyst crystal to hold and placed my large crystal wand beside me. I hoped I'd be able to concentrate better than I had that morning. Tomorrow would come soon enough. Then I would know about the lump in my breast.

I awoke down and depressed, but without a headache. I had hoped to ride Cadok and Robbie, but my heart wasn't in it. I was too tired. I thought back over the past days. I had pushed myself. I had believed I could build myself up by sheer physical effort. Ride two horses, organize Zuleika Farm West, attend the horse show, get the girls together for their photography session, do all the numerous things I managed to push into my day. Calculating that I had only two good weeks of energy and relaxation between chemos, I tried to make the most of them. I had decided those two good weeks would be used to whip me into shape, something to build on after my next treatment and the ensuing first week of nausea. But I had made no allowance for the fact that I was recovering from a serious illness and major surgery, not to mention the stress of living with disease and chemotherapy. I had fallen into my old patterns.

This Monday I would not leave the house until two o'clock to see Dr. Karlan. I tried to relax until then. But it was hard to turn off my motor. How did one pamper oneself? I had tea and toast. I couldn't bring myself to go back to bed. I leafed nervously through catalogues. Christmas editions were arriving, and it was only September 25. I marked ads for gifts. Then I remembered how draining Christmas was for me — all the gifts I gave to relatives, co-workers, staff and friends. Last year I had personally picked out three hundred gifts, all different, all chosen to fit the individual. For two months before Christmas my desk and surrounding floor space were covered with gifts, wrapping paper, ribbons, cards, lists, lists and lists. I determined not to burden myself this year. My children and close family would each receive only one gift. Friends would get a card. Surely, they would understand. I became tense again thinking about Christmas — in September, for crying out loud!

It was one o'clock, an hour before I had to be at Mitchell

Karlan's office. Goddammit, I hated being sick. I felt caged again. Trapped. Hate it, hate it! "Goddamn, goddamn," I repeated to myself. I was furious, fed up with my body and its fatigue. I decided to meditate. I found my tape player and headset. I closed the bedroom door, settled down and closed my eyes. After twenty minutes of good meditation I did feel better. Trying to hold on to the calm feeling, I ate a salad.

I went upstairs, put on a jumpsuit, no bra, no right tit. Why put on the prosthesis? I'd soon be taking it off again. Charlie said that in my straw hat and gray cotton, crop-legged jumpsuit I looked like a Japanese gardener. I thought I looked more like a rice planter in an old Japanese movie. Slipping my prosthesis into my large, woven rope beach bag in case we decided to go somewhere after the doctor's, I sprayed myself liberally with violet-scented cologne, then slid into the Jaguar next to Charlie and off we went.

20

MITCHELL KARLAN'S WAITING ROOM was crowded as usual. I caught some interesting stares as Charles Bronson barged in, hand in hand with his Japanese gardener. I wished I had my right tit in place instead of in my purse. Oh well, too late now. After a while the nurse announced my full name — Jill Bronson — confirming my identity for the curious. She put me in an examination room.

I stripped and held a small towel against myself. Within seconds, Mitch came briskly into the room. "Hi, how are you?"

"I'm worried. I have another lump."

I showed him exactly where it was. He closed his eyes and felt the area. "I'll have to give you a job, Jill. You're developing good fingers."

"Can you feel it?"

"Of course I can. It feels like a cyst; but, here, lie down. I'm going to give you a shot of Novocain."

Immediate panic. "Oh, no, don't do that." I covered my breast with my hand.

"If I don't aspirate it, Jill, you'll have to undergo surgery. I'll have to do a biopsy."

"Can you X-ray it?"

"Honey, if I don't get some fluid, you'll never know."

"Okay," I said, nearly in tears, "but ask Charlie to come in and hold my hand."

"You want him in here?"

"Yes, I do."

"Okay." He left for a second and returned. I was red-hot and my hands were sweating. Charlie came around to my right side and held me. I burst into tears. He stroked my head and put his lips against my temple.

"I'm sorry. I've lost all my courage."

Charlie had his face close to mine. "I wish I could do it for you," he said.

I felt Mitch wipe my breast with an alcohol swab while I cried. "I'm sorry, I'm so nervous. I'm sorry." But I wasn't sorry. I wanted to cry; it helped me.

In went the needle to draw out fluid. Mitch did it quickly, then held the syringe up to the light.

"God love you, it's okay. It's just a cyst. I hit one perfectly and got the fluid. It's fine. Look, it's clear. I don't even have to send it to the lab." He squirted the fluid down the sink. "Only one in a million comes back malignant when the fluid is clear. We've stopped bothering to have it tested if we pull clear fluid. If it were cancerous, the fluid would be bloody."

I wiped my eyes on the modesty towel, leaving smudges of blue kohl. "Thank you, Mitch, I'm so relieved."

He applied a Band-Aid. I put on my bra and right breast. Mitch smiled and said, "Congratulations. See you in three weeks."

Charlie and I hotfooted it out of there and went — where else? — to Neiman-Marcus. My limbs were moving as if I were pushing them along under water. I clung to Charlie. As we entered the elegant store, I asked, "Where do you want to go? What do you want to look at?"

"Let's look at hats," he said. "That's what you need right now."

We found a multitude of brightly colored felts, berets, trilbies. It was a lovely sight. Charlie was attracted by a beaded cloche. "How about this, Jill? You have a well-shaped head. It would look great on you."

It was very pretty. A gold-beaded skullcap with a beaded

fringe all around the neck and face. He was right — it did look good on me. He bought two, one gold, one bronze. My mind flashed to a little girl Jill listening to her father talk about his favorite sister, Elsie. Her husband used to tell Daddy, when Auntie Elsie was feeling down, "Jack, there's nothing wrong with her a new hat won't cure." Charlie must have subscribed to the same philosophy. Like my uncle, he was right. I did begin to feel better. He also picked a few berets for me to wear during the day — in blue to match the kohl around my eyes, black, cream and an alarming, shocking pink that I helped choose for the sheer courage of the color.

Charlie then sat me in a big, comfortable leather chair. So much had been riding on that single, small moment when the needle came out with clear liquid, I was exhausted. The relief hadn't really hit me yet.

Charlie told me, "Of course you're tired, baby. It was all the tension. That's what it was all about last night with the headache. It's as if you've been holding your own weight above your head."

I found that mental picture appropriate — using all my muscular skill to hold myself in the air — and now my muscles were tired. Charlie left me sitting in the reclining chair watching television while he prowled the men's department. I watched him. He tried on a black leather jacket and then put it back. He drifted to some hats and ties, then briefly looked at shirts. His face was kind and concerned. I could see his mind wasn't really on shopping. He was giving me time to rest and regroup. I looked at Charlie and thought how much I loved and needed him. It would be very nice to crawl into his pocket and stay there until I felt better.

As we drove home under a gray, stormy ceiling, I recalled Bernard Dowson saying, "I don't think you need a biopsy. As far as I can see, the cancer is gone." I realized my visit to Mitch had been a test of a sort in my relationship with Bernard. Bernard had passed with flying colors. At home, we dropped my hatboxes on the floor, went upstairs and lay on the bed. Charlie held me quietly. As I rested with my head on his shoulder, I knew it was the best place in the world.

I visited Sue Colin the following day. We discussed how fear had exhausted me and brought on the terrible headache on Monday. "You should have asked it what it had come to tell you," Sue suggested. She said a Valium was one way of dealing with it. But a better way would have been to ask the headache what it was there to tell me, and what I could do about it. I wished I had thought of that. I realized how powerful the human mind is, how devious and cunning. I really hadn't acknowledged all that fear. I had had the lump two weeks, but the anxiety had stayed in my subconscious until the last three days, when fatigue set in, followed by the headache. I left Sue Colin feeling more energized, more myself.

By four that afternoon my headache had snuck back. This time, I asked it what it wanted, why it had come. I immediately knew the answer; I should take a rest and some food. I did. I had my tea and rice bread with honey. Zuleika came in from school and, for once, I let Charlie take her to the stables, while I remained on my couch sticking snapshots in my summer photograph album. Don't push it, I thought. When you're tired, you're tired. You can't force yourself out of it. Just give in. Relax. Charlie loves spending time with Zuleika. She won't love you less for not going with her. Learn to delegate. My headache slipped away.

I carefully peeled the Band-Aid off my breast. I still wasn't really in touch with what a close call I'd had. Intellectually, yes, but my gut hadn't got the message. I think my subconscious took it, wrapped it up and tucked it away in a dark corner until I was ready to assimilate it. Yes, that lump, the size of a grape, had rattled my cage.

Valentine sent me a lovely, big bunch of flowers on Wednesday with a card: "I love you, Mom — from the Great One, Val." Valentine had called himself "Valentine the Great" since he was six, when he signed everything in his room, "Val the Great." *Val the Great* read his bedside lamp, *Val the Great* cried his headboard, *Val the Great* was the new signature in the corner of all the paintings in his room. He was right, of course — Val *is* great. We decided to put a crimp in his sails, however, when he started signing the dining room wallpaper. But since then, he has always been Val the Great to Charlie and me.

Jason, my blue-eyed, black-haired, gypsy son, called every night to see how my day had been and to say, "Good night, Mom, I love you." To my immense relief, Jason was facing things better now. Charlie, having intimately shared the moment of truth with me, was a mirror reflection of my feelings. When I felt good, he seemed happy, and when I was down, he was quiet and withdrawn.

I now had four days before my fifth chemo. Thursday was very up. I awoke feeling well, luxuriated in bed, went to the stable just for the privilege of visiting the horses.

Afterward, I got in my car, turned the radio to KHJ and sang at the top of my voice along with all the recent pop songs as I sped down Pacific Coast Highway, then along the freeway to Robertson Boulevard to my appointment with Sue Colin. Sue was pleased by my energy. She asked me to list all the gifts that cancer had brought me. This is my list:

1. Getting a beach house.
2. Independence.
3. More confidence.
4. More at ease with myself. More assertive.
5. Taking time to grow.
6. Writing. I had always wanted to write, but had never given myself the time. Now I not only found the time, but I also had a subject that I really wanted to write about.
7. My marriage had become even closer.
8. I was doing more of my own thing, living more of my own life.
9. It had helped me to be myself
10. It had brought meditation to my life.
11. It had made me conscious of my health and encouraged me to eat a more sensible diet.

12. It had enriched my relationships with my children and the people close to me.

Sue wrote the list for me and looked at it. "These are a lot of goodies, Jill. Do you think you've got enough? Are you ready to give up your cancer now?"

I knew what she meant. Cancer had been the answer to a lot of things. I thought about it further. It had given me the courage to do what I really needed to do rather than what was expected of me.

"I hope I am, Sue. I really hope so. When I found the lump in my left breast, I certainly became very angry. For somebody who's not ready to give up cancer, I certainly have been fighting hard. I'm aware there could be something going on in my deeper subconscious, something that isn't quite ready to give it up. But I think I am prepared to do so. I hope so."

God, I hoped so.

I was still in a wonderfully good mood. Sue had lead crystal in different shapes hanging from cords in her window. The sun came in at different times to create rainbows in the room. I liked to try to catch them in my hand. I spent the remaining time with Sue doing just that. All of a sudden, there was a pounding at the door.

"Who's that?" I asked.

"It's the next person," Sue replied.

I said good-bye and made an appointment for the following Wednesday. She said, "Why don't you come in Monday morning before your chemotherapy? You're not having it until three. I can relax you before you go."

"No, I think it's better that I do luxurious things that please me. Maybe I'll go to the barn or write or sit home and read or just walk my dog. I'm going to do relaxing things." I didn't want to make the drive to town twice. I said good-bye and left.

I had left my car at a wash to have it waxed and the windows tinted. It looked splendid, all shiny, good as new with its tinted windows. I hopped in and drove cheerily home, once again singing at the top of my lungs. I really enjoyed driving these days, and I loved listening to the radio blasting out the hits.

I also began laughing again. Really laughing. For three months I'd been a rather solemn person. My eyes were serious. I could see it when I put the photographs in my album. Certainly, I would laugh with my friends and family, but it didn't come from my heart. Now, laughter was breaking through, rather like tulips coming up in spring. I had frozen my feelings. Now it seemed spring was coming in September. Little things Charlie said made me laugh. When we discussed remodeling the new house, he said, "What I'm really looking forward to is a nice, big dressing room of my own. If we share a bathroom and dressing room, you'll put your things all over the place. My side will be cluttered with your possessions. I won't have anywhere to put my stuff." This made me laugh. I also cried easily. For months I had tried to be stoic; but, now, when something happened, I was so in touch with my feelings I burst into tears like a child. Laughter and tears came easily for me, and it was most pleasant.

Sunday was a fun day. I went to the stable. Zuleika had brought a friend, Rachel, home from the horse show, so they came along, too. I rode my old friend Cadok. Zuleika and Rachel hit the trails with two of Zuleika's horses, her Connemara, Turtle, and her jumper, Loppy. I didn't think about tomorrow much at all. As usual, the horses kept me in the moment.

In the evening we were to have dinner with friends. I raided my wardrobe for something for Katrina to wear, as all her going-out-to-dinner clothes were at the Bel Air house. It was fun dressing her up. Zuleika, being younger, thought she could get away with faded blue jeans and a shirt of mine that she had had her eye on. We drove down the coast to a gourmet French restaurant where, indeed, everyone was rather formally attired.

We joined a young producer and his actress wife. He had

telephoned a few weeks earlier to say he was in the same situation I was; he had cancer. He'd told me of the wonderful doctor he was seeing, and I'd told him about Bernard Dowson and Sue Colin. I had asked how he handled the fear and he'd replied that he couldn't talk about it. I was the first person, apart from his wife, with whom he had discussed his illness. I urged him then to seek therapy to help him handle the fear. Our dinner was ostensibly for business, but I was seated next to him and, of course, *the* subject came up. I told him how helpful therapy had been for me. He said his wife would be away for two weeks on a movie location. He had recently undergone surgery and thought perhaps he wouldn't go with her; instead, he would take the two weeks to start seeing Bernard. He was reluctant to see a therapist, too scared to pull out the stops and open the dam, as he put it. I felt I shouldn't push. But I thought what he really needed was to see Sue Colin, or someone else he could relate to. The fear is so terrible to live with.

At dinner, the girls were enchanting and his wife, charming. We saw Walter Matthau in the restaurant. He had grown a long, rabbinical beard and looked unusual, to say the least. He was with his wife and the director Billy Wilder and his wife. As we left, both Walter's and Billy's wives waved to us gaily. We waved back. My fine handkerchief linen dress floated around my ankles. In my pretty new gold-beaded hat, I felt quite elegant.

I slept well that night in spite of being full of exquisite French cooking and wine, which I wasn't supposed to have. I had also allowed myself a raspberry daiquiri — they didn't have strawberry. I meditated, but I was so sleepy it was hard to concentrate.

I awoke the next morning with no feeling of foreboding or tension. I meditated, then went downstairs to have breakfast with Charlie. My husband is the most disciplined man I've ever known, the most disciplined *person* I've ever known. Every morning after his coffee, without fail, he goes upstairs to exercise. We spend our mornings independently and it works well. This morning, I answered my correspondence, went through my bills, signed a few checks, took the dog for a walk and ate scrambled eggs on toast. I was relaxed. I wasn't scared of the approaching chemotherapy. I really knew what to expect now. Charlie and I were going to leave the house at two o'clock. I wasn't even watching the clock.

When we got to Michael's office I strode boldly in. No crying in the corner this time. I walked to the desk where Michael stood with his two receptionists.

"Hi, Jill. Come right in."

I had my blood test, and Michelle said, "You can come right in now, Jill." I asked Charlie to join us.

Michelle is a slender, brown-haired woman in her middle thirties with nice blue eyes that crinkle when she smiles. She has an important quality, a good sense of humor.

"How are you feeling?" she asked.

"Not bad."

"You don't look so hot."

"Well, Michelle, I've decided it's easier not to try to be cheerful and up. I just go with my feelings. It takes tremendous energy to deal with all this, and I can't afford to spend any trying to be amusing when I don't feel like it."

She said, "No, that's fine."

However, I found myself saying funny things all the same. Charlie and Michelle were a good audience. I kept them laughing until Michael came in.

"Your blood test is okay, so let's get on with it," he said.

Michelle plopped the ice helmet on my head after first tourniqueting my brow. Soon I was getting my IV injection. This time I sat up, which made me feel less vulnerable, less "take me, I'm yours-ish."

I asked Michelle, "Are you sure I can take the chemo sitting up?" The first day I asked, Michael had told me, "No, if you sit up, all the veins get bent."

Michelle said, "I've never heard anything so ridiculous in my life," so we proceeded with me sitting up. It was quite a jolly treatment as treatments go.

I told Michelle how on Saturday I had walked into a hairdresser's, sat down, given the girl a bottle of tint and told her to fix my hair, saying, "Just put this on, dear, and don't worry about the bald spots — I'm having chemotherapy."

The poor girl couldn't say anything for thirty minutes.

Michelle found the story amusing, so I told her how I had imagined, when my hair was falling out, going to a beauty shop for a shampoo just to see the shock on the poor girl's face as my hair came out in handfuls. Michelle said, "Oh, you're wicked."

Then I cried out, "Oh, Michelle, I can feel it, I can feel it! Stop." The needle burned my arm. She told me to open and close my fist a few times, which I did. But there was no relief. "It still hurts, Michelle."

"Keep opening and closing your fist, Jill. That's right. Does it feel any better?"

"Oh, a little." The three vials of chemicals went in slowly. God bless Michelle. It was the first time I had taken therapy without holding Charlie's hand. I was handling it better. Michael came in as we finished.

I made an appointment for my two-week blood check, and we drove home. I wasn't feeling too bad; in fact, I felt well enough that evening to eat two slices of pizza — a real no-no. That, combined with dinner at the French restaurant the night before, should really have made me sick, but the pizza looked so good I couldn't resist. I hadn't seen Bernard Dowson for some time now and it seemed that with Bernard away, the mouse will play.

I ran a warm bubble bath, taking my usual long look at myself in the mirror before I stepped into the tub. "Well, you don't look so bad, old girl," I said to myself. "Now it has to be qualititty, not quantitty." Ha, ha. I sank into the warm water, definitely feeling cocky. Chemotherapy number five was over. Yea, me! Five down, three to go. I'd broken the back, I'd passed the halfway mark. I enjoyed my bath, wrapped myself in a blue bathrobe and went downstairs to study the four stones on the coffee table.

"Which one shall I throw, Charlie?"

"The big one."

"But it's so attractive."

He came over and studied them. "This one. It looks like a sore." There was no further decision to be made. I picked up the "sore," went out on the veranda and hurled the rock as far as I could into the ocean. The tide had come in and the sea was swirling in the pilings under the house, so this wasn't difficult. Charlie stood beside me. "Maybe you should have let me throw it, so it won't get washed back."

"Charlie! I threw it far enough."

He laughed. "Sure you did, baby. You did."

I was feeling obnoxiously well. I went upstairs and uncovered the wig. So far, it hadn't gone anywhere. I put it on, went back downstairs and watched TV for the rest of the evening. I was beginning to feel queasy. The queasiness was accompanied by the red-hot feeling. I saw it out, meditated and went to bed. I curled up with my head on Charlie's shoulder until I was sleepy enough to turn onto my left side and sleep. My last words to myself were directed at my blood cells: "Okay, guys, come on, you know what this is about. We've done it before. You can handle it. You know you're not supposed to take it in. I'm doing this for the good of my body. Everything's cool. We made it. We're going to sleep now. Good night."

I awoke the next morning feeling frail. I spent a quiet day, mostly lying on my couch. It was as if I were running alternately a high fever and freezing chills. Later in the afternoon Charlie and I visited the House That Jack Built. Once again, as I walked around the house, I had a good, warm feeling. This was, indeed, the home for me. The rest of the day was spent resting.

The following day my energy improved. Charlie was in town for a meeting, so Alan stopped by to take me for a cheerful lunch at La Scala. I gorged on Italian food, but I had no nausea afterward. Alan was panicked about Bernard Dowson. He hadn't been able to contact him for almost two weeks. I had received a call from his receptionist, telling me there was a family emergency and Bernard would be gone until the first of the month. Alan was stunned.

"How can he leave you? How can he leave all his patients who need him?"

I hadn't had a treatment on the table in two weeks. It seemed I wouldn't be getting another for a long time. I missed my two visits a week and the reassurance from the electromagnetic waves coursing through my body, killing cancer cells.

Alan called Bernard daily, leaving messages on his answering machine. I ran out of little brown bottles of electrically charged water. I ran out of the vitamins Bernard had given me. I had a vague, uneasy feeling all was not well.

The premonition was confirmed when I visited Sue Colin. She said, "The American Medical Association cracked down on Bernie. Homeopathic healers are not allowed to dispense." Somebody reported Bernard for selling vitamins. I told Sue I thought something like that had happened. She said, "It makes me so mad. He helps people. He gets results."

In this country, homeopathic doctors are not allowed to diagnose, which Bernard didn't do in my case. I went to him with my own diagnosis.

She told me, "President Reagan uses a homeopathic doctor."

I agreed, "So do the Queen of England and Prince Charles." I wondered when I would be able to go back and have my treatments.

Sue said Bernard might be able to see me in a couple of weeks. I now knew I really wanted to get back on that table soon. I wanted the best of all worlds: the AMA, my homeopathic healer, and my holistic therapists. They were all important.

21

NOT LONG AFTER MY FIFTH chemotherapy session, Alan again broached the subject of reconstructive surgery. He'd found a wonderful plastic surgeon. I still didn't want an implant. I had an image of myself living to sixty or seventy with one drooped left tit and one pert, young, right one. Alan said, "You'd have to have them both done."

"Well, that would mean I'd have to take the left one off and start again. I'm not going to do that if I can help it." That set me thinking about Las Vegas show girls. What happened when their bodies aged and they became old women? Did they still have two young breasts? The idea seemed ludicrous. I would have to think hard and long before replacing that right breast.

By Wednesday, I was still tired and draggy. Alan had finally contacted Bernard through Judith, his receptionist. I made an appointment for two weeks' time. Bernard sent me a brown bottle of drops, which were supposed to be very powerful, to make up for missing the electromagnetic table treatments. That day was spent on my couch, surrounded by my favorite cures. I drank glasses and glasses of watermelon juice and water to flush my system effectively. I knew some people smoked marijuana to get them through postchemotherapy nausea. I didn't try it, but I did find that curry powder introduced into my food, usually as a sauce over fresh vegetables, somehow helped sort out my stomach. So I ate curry, drank watermelon juice and at least ten glasses of water a day. I took my drops from Bernard — ten drops four times a day — and waited.

I was weary of waiting. I had been a semi-invalid for two years. I wondered if I would ever feel fit and well again. I wanted to run as fast as I could. I wanted to ride a strong, good-moving horse, to gallop over fields and jump fences. I was feeling sorry for myself. So, another glass of watermelon juice, turn on the tape and meditate, put my nose back to the grindstone, the grindstone of getting well.

God, sometimes I was a bore. I knew I was fortunate financially. I was having the deluxe version of the disease. I was so grateful to have people to help me pack, move, take care of my horses and homes. I was grateful we could afford to pay Dino's and Antonio's salaries so that domestic duties could be delegated. I was thankful we could afford all the things I was doing in my quest for health. How different things would have been without the financial resources available to me. When I think how hard it could have been, I shudder.

Cancer wipes out families financially, changes life-styles, destroys plans and hopes and dreams. Life had been kind to me, I know.

Still, I slipped into desperation. I felt miserably angry, trapped. Once I spent an entire day eating. I ate everything I could think of — things I should eat, things I should not eat. I felt unattractive. I wanted to have long, silky, blond hair. I wanted two breasts. I wanted something to look forward to. I was angry, but I didn't know with whom or what to be angry. I had been so looking forward to the new house. Now, with problems in negotiating the contract and escrow, I wondered if we shouldn't look for another house. We were spending so much money. Was the House That Jack Built really what we wanted? Maybe there were negative things we wouldn't discover until after we bought the place.

I wanted to jump in my car and drive away as fast as I

could — but to what? To where? Perhaps I should get into bed, curl up and pull the covers over my head. No, too boring. No one told me cancer would be so boring.

My boredom was temporarily relieved one day when Valentine came to visit us with Marty, one of his friends. Valentine wore a troubled expression, the kind that usually meant he wanted a private conversation with Charlie. But I wasn't disposed to leave my couch, so I asked, "What's the matter? You look worried."

"Well, Mom, it's not something I want to talk about with you." He glanced momentarily at Marty. Marty stared at the floor; he didn't want anything to do with whatever it was.

"Oh, come on, Valentine; you've got to tell us now. Charlie, tell him to tell us."

Valentine put on a brave front. With a wry smile on his already sheepish face, he told us, "I've got *crabs!*"

"WHAT!" I screamed. "Get up off that chair this instant. Eyuu! Crabs!"

Val jumped off the chair, then, seeing I was hysterical with laughter, he sat down again. I couldn't stop laughing.

"Jesus, Val," said Charlie. "Who gave you those? Not Pesty?"

"No, I haven't been seeing Pesty recently."

I tried to control my mirth. "Val, I'm sorry I'm laughing, but it's such a surprise."

Marty looked brighter now that he saw how we were taking the news.

"Val," I asked, "what are you doing about them?"

"Well, I went to see Dr. Weston because I was scratching and itching so badly, then I found this thing."

"This what?" I shrieked.

"This crab thing. Here, you want to see one?" He put his hands down his pants and made as if to pull something out to show me.

I screamed, "God, no, Val!"

He laughed. "I don't have them anymore. Ray gave me this shampoo. It's supposed to get rid of them."

By now I was hysterical again. "Well, darling, I don't know where you got them, but I hope you can figure it out and not go back for more. Maybe you should wear a flea collar around your neck and around your you-know-what!"

"Mom!"

Charlie asked, "What did Ray say, Val?"

Val laughed. "Well, Dr. Weston got this magnifying glass and was peering at me. I told him, 'Watch out, Doctor, don't get your beard too close, those little devils jump!' God, Charlie, I was scratching for days before I figured out what was wrong. Now, Mom, I know you think this is very funny, but I don't, so please don't tell anyone."

"Okay, Val, but you won't mind if I write it in my book, will you?"

Val was horrified. "What! You'd write about that?"

"Don't worry, Val, I'll simply write, 'Val came to visit us one day with his friend Marty, who had crabs.' "

It was Marty's turn to look uncomfortable. "Now, wait a minute," he said.

Laughing, I said, "Yes, that's what I'll do. I'll say Val's friend Marty, who lives at — where do you live, Marty? — has crabs, and my son Val, who was the last person you'd expect to have a friend with crabs, said . . ."

Marty and Val were laughing now. "Okay, Mom, okay. I'm going for a swim."

"Don't use any of our towels," I cautioned.

I felt better for the belly laugh. Three months later Val finally broke down and said it was okay if I wrote about him, but with the proviso that I preface the incident with "Val was the last person you'd expect to have something like crabs, because he is such a clean person." Then he had laughed and said, "No, that's okay. You say what you like."

"Never mind about the towels, Val, I love you, crabs and all." I gave him a big hug.

"Mom, I don't have crabs anymore!" Val said as he and Marty turned to leave the room.

"I know darling, and you're not the first or last person

to have had them." I made a crawly motion with my hand.
"Mom!"

I jumped a foot in the air, aimed at his face and kissed him.
"I love you, Val. I'll never mention crabs again." My six-foot
seven-inch son walked stiffly from the room, pausing just long
enough in the door frame to turn to me and scratch fever-
ishly. "Remember the flea collars, Val," I called after him.

The next day, Jason phoned.

"Happy anniversary, Mom."

"What? What anniversary? What are you talking about?"

"It's your wedding anniversary, isn't it, October fifth?"

"October fifth," I said in a daze. "Oh, yes. Hey, Charlie, it's
our wedding anniversary."

Charlie covered his face with his hands. "You're kidding?
Oh, God."

"Oh, well," I said, "we've been forgetting the date for the
last fifteen years. We wouldn't want to break with tradition."

Later, Charlie talked to the realtor on the phone. He told
me the deal was dead — we were not going to buy the House
That Jack Built after all. Well, I wasn't surprised. I was hardly
disappointed. I didn't feel much of anything.

"Oh, let's go out and eat a Mexican meal."

"You're not supposed to, it's not on your diet."

"I don't care. It's our anniversary. I want Mexican food."

We ate a large Mexican meal. I drank a glass of white wine,
which didn't go well at all. It made me sick. Even so, I continued to eat throughout the evening. I was packing food
into my body to see how much I could stuff in, as if I were a
sausage. Charlie tenderly rubbed my belly, saying, "My little
pig." I had been eating almost nonstop for three days. I
wished I could stop. It made me uncomfortable, but that was
what I wanted to do — eat.

At one point, I felt as if I were going to split wide open. I
crammed in everything I could think of. One moment I decided I would ask Sue Colin if she could hypnotize me out of
this eating binge. A split second later I ate a quarter of a bag

of Famous Amos chocolate chip cookies. I hadn't had a cookie in two months. The sugar gave me quite a high. I had bought myself a bright orange army surplus flight suit, loose and comfortable. I put it on and settled down on my couch. Charlie's little pig decided to munch the rest of the weekend away. I couldn't fight it, so I might as well enjoy it. Munch, munch, munch.

During meditation that night, when it came to the part where I imagined my white blood cells doing their job, I formed a mental image of myself as one of the cells. I was at the head of a pack of sharklike fish, representing the cells. They had large, sharp fangs. I joined them in gnashing my teeth on a large tumor. I could hear the sound of smacking teeth around me, slashing and ripping. I began to bite my teeth together as I meditated. I clenched my fist and pounded on the chair, full of energy, determination and rage. I was happy with the imagery of flashing teeth slurping, smacking and biting into the cancerous tumor. I completed meditating and, satisfied with myself, went to sleep.

The following evening Charlie, languid as a cat, eyes golden, slightly brooding, watched me as we entertained friends for dinner at La Scala. I wore white crepe jodhpurs, and a white silk shirt over which I had put a man's dark gray pin-striped frock coat. On my head I wore a black bowler. My riding cronies were there, Kathy Kuzner, Susie Dotan and Pesty and Valentine. We had fun at the table. I'd bounced back. My depression was over.

On Monday, a full week after chemo five, I had clicked over and felt like my old self.

"Let's take a walk, Charlie. Let's do a couple of miles."

I got into my shorts, T-shirt and running shoes. We did two fourteen-minute miles, the first of our walks since my surgery. I was striding out, swinging my arms, chest uplifted, or at least half of it was uplifted. I strode down the road with Charlie and Cassie flanking me. It was a beautiful day. My body could handle the speed at which I traveled. It was a wonderful feeling. I had believed I would never do this again, and here I was doing it. I kept saying to Charlie, "I feel so happy I'm doing this."

Later that day, I went to the stable and rode Cadok. Feeling up as I was, I decided to put him over his first jump since his vanning accident. I had Sue Overholt set a low horizontal pole about half a foot off the ground. When Cadok saw the jump he pricked up his ears. I could feel his body coming together beneath me as I trotted him toward it, almost as if he were saying, "A jump — she thinks I can jump." We trotted toward the fence. Cadok jumped. He stumbled a little on landing, but immediately recovered. He snorted and cantered on.

"He can jump, Sue. He can actually get his hind end off the ground. Raise the pole a little." We trotted around again. Sue raised the pole; once again Cadok managed to jump. I patted him. "We're doing okay, buddy. We're going to be all right." I gave him his bath. He seemed pleased with himself. It was a new beginning for both of us.

A little disappointment was at hand, however. I became aware of pressure under my right armpit and, by the time I got home, it was quite uncomfortable. I undressed and raised my arm to find three lumps distending the skin. I recognized the problem as phlebitis. I had encountered it about four weeks after surgery. I thought this time it was probably due to my brisk walks and arm-swinging. I was angry. I didn't want anything to come between me and walking and riding. But thanks somewhat to the good bottle of Marqués de Riscal we had at dinner, I managed to put the anger aside. I slept that night with my arm on a pillow beside me, my one concession to the problem.

22

"WELL," SUE SAID AT MY appointment the following morning, "what's up?"

I shrugged. "I'm worried about a condition in the area of my surgery. I have this phlebitis in my armpit that runs down to my elbow. I can't lift my arm and I feel as if somebody applied a tourniquet under my armpit. I'm sure it's caused by my walks, but I don't want to stop. I don't want to give in to it."

Sue said, "I can't believe you, Jill. You're always the same. Your body is telling you it needs rest. You've pushed it too far."

"But, Sue, it's so frustrating. I just begin to make progress and something happens. I begin to feel happy that I can build on what I've started — my walking — and something puts me down."

"I know it's difficult, but you must listen to your body. Your body never lies. It's telling you now to rest. You're not healed enough."

"But, Sue, it's been three months."

"Nevertheless, it's too soon."

"I'm so frustrated, so angry. The rest of my body enjoys walking. The rest of me can handle it."

"But a part of you can't. Now it's speaking to you. Do you want to wait until it screams at you?"

Giving in to physical incapacity has always been difficult for me. No one in my family gives in. My husband is such a strong person, physically and mentally, it's hard for him to realize someone else can break. I fell and hurt my leg once when we were skiing. Charlie said, "Get up and give it a shake; it'll probably be all right." I tried, but it wasn't all right. However, determined to tough it out, I held on to someone's ski poles and skied down the mountain, which took thirty minutes. My leg was broken and I walked with crutches for four months.

Everybody thought I handled it rather well. When it was necessary for me to use crutches, I wrapped bright, colorful ribbons around them to match all my outfits. At least I did with my first broken leg. With my third leg fracture — I broke my limbs regularly — snap, snap, snap — I didn't bother with ribbons, but I always made sure I dressed more attractively than usual in outfits to accommodate the casts and iron braces. I have always been accident-prone. Maybe that's why I am good at graceful recoveries. At times, I thought I did better as an invalid than as a whole person.

Before my surgery, I had depleted my system, using up more and more energy from my quota, until finally I was using energy constantly, stressing myself, ignoring my need to replenish. I abandoned my outlets. I hadn't worked as an actress for two years. Injuries prevented me from riding. I was left running the horse business in California and Vermont, and business was not good. It was a strain. The two homes were a hassle. There was the underlying panic of a leg that wouldn't heal. Then, when Katrina's mother, Hilary, died, I had no free, private time. I was nurturing Katrina and it wasn't enough; Katrina, justifiably, needed more. At the same time, determined not to take anything away from my Zuleika, I gave myself even more to her. I gave and stretched, trying to spread my arms out as far as they would go. Then, when they weren't enough, I stretched my fingers.

Finally, my body gave me another smack. It had been warning me all year with headaches, backaches, sleepless nights and the ailing leg. Now it launched a frontal attack —

breast cancer. "Listen!" it screamed. Now, at last, I was listening.

At first I couldn't see how I was going to be able to change. I resisted Dr. Simonton's efforts to tell me I had to change. I rationalized everything.

Now Sue asked me to think back to all the injuries and illnesses I could remember. The question made me think of Simonton's book, in which he asks readers to reflect on all the illnesses they have suffered in their lives, and the events preceding and surrounding them. So I took a trip down memory lane, recalling incidents and illnesses from childhood through my teens and twenties.

I recalled an ice-skating accident when I was thirteen. I was kicked in the leg by another skater. I spent six weeks in bed with that injury, and discovered my allergy to penicillin. When I was eighteen, dancing with the Monte Carlo Ballet Company, I tore all the ligaments in my right ankle. The ballet mistress soaked my ankle in ice, numbing it, and I danced that night, weakening it forever, ruining my chance of becoming a serious dancer. During a one-year period when I was nineteen I had three car accidents. One ruined my ankle and another hospitalized me for two months, ending my plum role in an important movie. Professional suicide, Bill Watts, my agent at the time, had called it in a telegram he sent to the hospital.

Then my mind drifted back to my fourth pregnancy.

Paul was two years old. After his birth I became pregnant twice, both times miscarrying. Now I was being given shots to help me carry my fourth pregnancy to full term.

It was 1961 when David got a role in *The Great Escape*, to be filmed in Germany. We always needed money. As a good wife, I was to accompany him with Paul. I had been hospitalized for three weeks due to difficulties with my pregnancy. I left the hospital in a wheelchair to join David, Paul and my mother (who was going along to help) in David's speedy Jaguar.

It was a long drive to Munich involving a ferry across the

147

English Channel and a route through Germany's Black Forest. On the autobahn through the Black Forest David braked to a screeching halt. He was traveling at maybe ninety-five to one hundred miles an hour when a huge buck deer leaped out on the highway. We barely avoided hitting it. I braced myself by putting my feet up on the dashboard. I was thrown forward in the fetal position and felt a tremendous pressure and impact go through my body. Paul and my mother, in the backseat, were shocked and thrown around, but unhurt.

The next day, in the car as we were driving, my water broke. To avoid soiling the leather seats, I wrapped myself in a blanket as we drove through the dark night until we reached Munich. We hadn't planned to stay in that city, but I was in such a bad way — exhausted, weak and shaky — that David took two rooms at the Four Seasons Hotel.

The following day was June 2, a prophetic date, Paul's birthday. I went to bed in the hotel while David and my mother took Paul down to the restaurant. I was left alone in the room. Lying in the dim light, I became aware of a presence in the room, a dark, shadowy figure standing behind my right shoulder. It was the figure of an Indian. It just stood there. I was comforted by its presence. I knew it was guarding me, just there to keep me company.

I never before had had an experience like that; I have never since. But it was a profound sense that I was not alone, that a patient, kindly being was there with me, caring for me. I was not at all frightened, only comforted. I needed guarding. We were in serious trouble, the baby and I. The baby had died (or was at that moment dying within me). I hadn't sensed it yet.

My family came back. I seemed to be okay. The water no longer leaked out of me. David decided we should relax for a day and then proceed on our journey to Posenhaufen, a lakeside town and our final destination. The next day I stayed in bed. We all thought I was fine. I wasn't bleeding, which had previously been cause for alarm throughout my pregnancy. I ordered a bottle of champagne. We had a glass to celebrate our arrival in Munich and Paul's third birthday. I let Paul have a glass, shocking my mother. Paul loved it. He and I giggled and laughed, having a really good time, me in bed and he sitting on it, enjoying the occasion.

The next day we traveled to Posenhaufen for a three-month location. I went to bed, to rest. But after a week I began bleeding. David found a doctor who spoke only German. We spoke only English and some French. He declared everything was *"sehr gut."* I trusted all doctors and so did David and my mother, so sehr gut we felt. He told me to continue bed rest, or at least we thought that's what he said. He put a stethoscope to my abdomen and listened. Then he indicated to David, while nodding approvingly, that he could also listen to the baby's heartbeat. With the help of a phrase book, we deduced he was leaving on a two-week vacation and would look in on me on his return. Okay. Sehr gut. I had the German medical seal of approval. My mother would stay on until I was able to resume my maternal duties. For now, I was to remain in bed.

Then it happened. Close to midnight, two weeks after the water broke, I went into labor. I was in great pain, but we pretended nothing was happening, hoping the pains would pass. Maybe it was gas or indigestion. My mother, hearing sounds of discomfort through the wall, came into the room to see what was happening. She recognized the situation. By now, I was in agony. She gave me a hairbrush to bite on. Now *I* knew what was happening. The pains were terrible and I recognized them. David rushed out for help. There was no one at the switchboard, so he drove from the hotel to find a doctor, a hospital, something. I was yelling, "Oh, God, help me. Someone, help me." Paul, hearing the din, came into my room. My mother, concerned for the child, took him to his room. While she was gone, I got out of bed. I squatted on the floor by the side of the bed and had a baby boy. We were alone, he and I. He was premature, a six-month delivery; he was not alive. I was barely living myself. I immediately began hemorrhaging. I was too weak to pull myself back up on the bed. I just sat on the floor with my little dead baby boy. The afterbirth hadn't yet delivered itself, but I was bleeding profusely.

At that moment my mother returned. She saw her daughter and grandchild in a bloody mess on the floor. "Oh, my God" was all she said.

I kept saying, "Oh, God, how awful. Oh, how awful."

My mother said, "It's not awful, darling, it's all right. Everything will be all right." She somehow got me back on the bed. Then David arrived with two ambulance men. I remember little of the drive to the hospital. I never saw my baby again.

I was put in Dr. Wilgruber's Krankenfrau Clinic for sick women. It was a maternity hospital as well. I was awakened the next morning by the sound of crying babies. I was in a large, bright room with one other bed. A motherly midwife-type nurse entered carrying a baby wrapped in a blue blanket. She came to me with an air of cozy importance. Smiling, she gave me the baby. Suddenly from the next bed came a torrent of German. The nurse snatched the baby from my arms and left the room. The woman in the next bed knew my story. She had seen me arrive the night before. Now she came to me and explained (in English, thank God) that the nurse had made a terrible mistake, that she had brought me someone else's baby. It was feeding time at the hospital, she explained, and the nurse had simply brought the baby into the wrong room.

Being a proper English girl, I controlled my desire to cry. I used my best manners and thanked the woman and introduced myself. We became friends for the six weeks I was to remain in the hospital.

During that time, I would get somewhat better, then when it seemed I could be discharged, I would hemorrhage. Blood would gush out of me, masses of it, accompanied by labor pains and the eventual delivery of huge blood clots, some almost the size of a two-pound fetus. This went on until I was in extremis. I had lost all the blood I could lose without dying. They couldn't give me blood as fast as I could lose it.

One day, through the haze of my agony, I realized I was dying.

Little Paul visited me every day. He looked so lonely and lost seeing his mother in bed in a strange place. To cheer him up, I drew faces on oranges. Paul wanted me to come home. He missed me. I knew I was in a life-and-death situation. I knew unless the bleeding was stopped I would die. I remember thinking, what a shame. I have a young child who needs me. What a shame. I'm dying.

Dr. Wilgruber took me into surgery one night. I don't know what he did. I guess it was a D and C and some repair work. Speaking only German, all he could say to me in English as I lay on the operating table awaiting the anesthetic was, "Exploration, not operation." He said it twice, very clearly. Thank God for those understanding words, "Exploration, no operation." I started to fight at that moment, just before they put me out. I now realize that it was my inner life force that took over. I urgently desired to be there for my son. I suddenly knew it was up to me and I started to fight just before the anesthetic took over. I now believe that that catastrophic illness, and all the others, was almost as if I were in training. It was to forge my understanding of pain and my ultimate ability to face this impossible, life-threatening situation.

To Sue, I said, "I seem to have been ill and accident-prone all my life. I remember walking home from school as a child in the rain and dawdling in puddles and becoming ill with sore throats and swollen glands." Then I repeated the story of my bout with Pinkus' disease when I was only ten months old.

"That's it, Sue, that's why I have so much patience when I'm ill. I had practice as a baby. I just sat there waiting in the glass case. It conditioned me for the rest of my life."

"Yes, you waited for someone to come along and pick you up and take care of you. Are you still doing that?"

"I don't know. I don't have any feelings on that subject. I don't have any feelings about it at all."

"Try to contact the feelings you *do* have. What do you feel while you are waiting?"

"Isolation. Cancer makes me feel isolated. I feel numb, nothingness."

"Do you like the feeling of nothingness, isolation and shutting down your feelings?"

"No, I don't, but it's worked well for me."

"Do you want to keep it?"

"No, I don't."

She told me to practice staying in touch with my feelings all the time, not to let myself daydream and drift into nothingness when I worried. To touch my sweater, be aware of how I felt, to rub my skin to see how it felt. It sounds easy, but I knew it would be difficult. I had become too expert at copping out by shutting down feelings whenever they became uncomfortable. I wondered what it was like to be aware of what you felt twenty-four hours a day. It sounded like hell. I had always been a daydreamer. Daydreaming protected me, muffled the screams of protest I heard in my head. I resolved to follow Sue's suggestion to keep myself in the present.

On the way home I gave thought to my long-held conviction that the world would stop if I changed and no longer performed as I had in the past. I smiled, recalling how Alan had yelled at me, "For God's sake, girl, if you die, everything and everyone will carry on. You know that. Nothing will stop."

I thought to myself, "It looks as if I have to die so that I can live."

It was clear to me now that certain lifelong behavior and convictions had to die so I could survive.

By the time the beach house loomed in sight, I had made up my mind. I would help myself. I would take more responsibility for wellness, not illness. I would *not* walk two miles today. I would visit Cadok, but not ride him. I would rest my arm. I telephoned Mitchell Karlan about the phlebitis. He said it was unusual that it should show up so long after surgery. He thought it had been brought on by my walks and

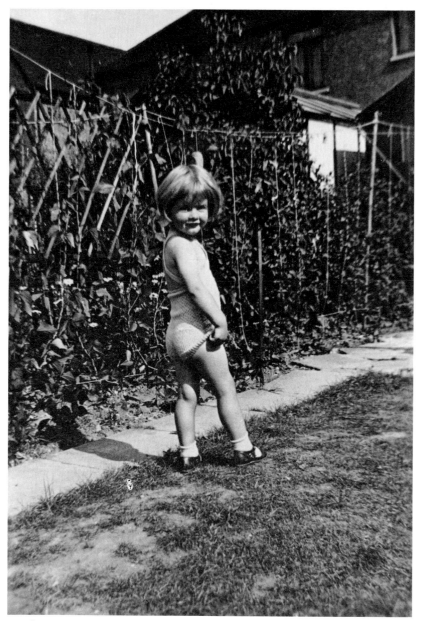

In the garden of my parents' house in England, age 2.

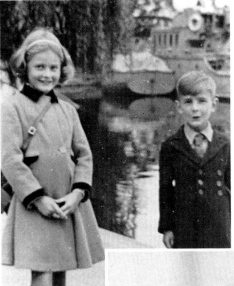

At age 8, with brother, John, 6, on Swan Walk, Richmond, England.

My grade school photograph at age 10.

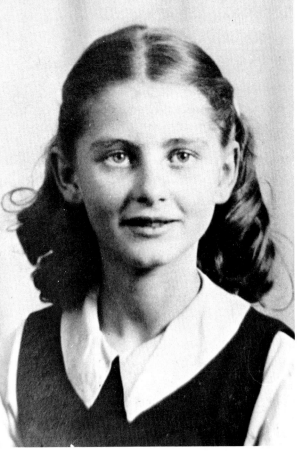

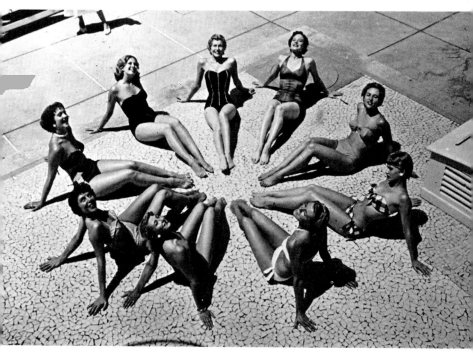

Here I am, in the black-and-white-checked bikini with members
of the Anita Avila ballet company, at the swimming pool of the
Monte Carlo Sporting Club, Monte Carlo, in 1954.

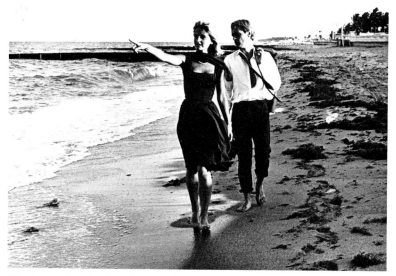

With my first husband, David McCallum, strolling on the
beach in Florida, 1963.

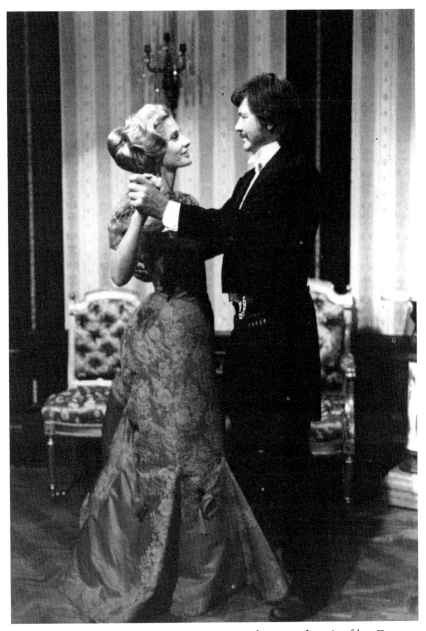

With Charles, in a romantic scene from my favorite film, From Noon Till Three. (Frankovich Productions)

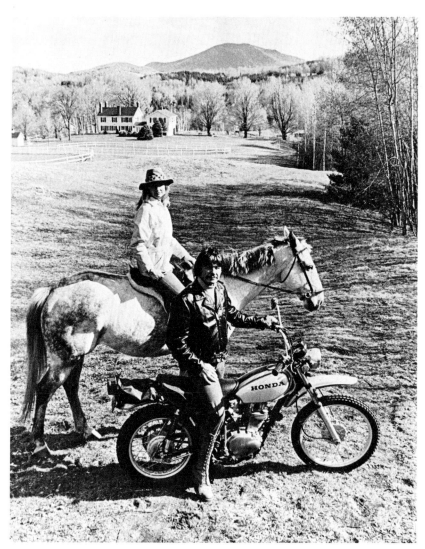

At Zuleika Farm in Vermont, in 1974, I am riding Dennis, my favorite horse at that time, and Charles is on his motor bike. (John Byrson)

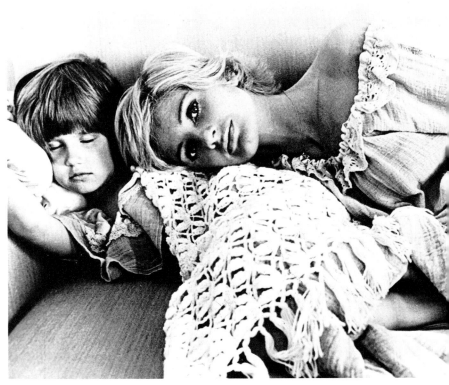

At the Cannes Film Festival, with Zuleika, age 4, in a moment of repose, 1975.

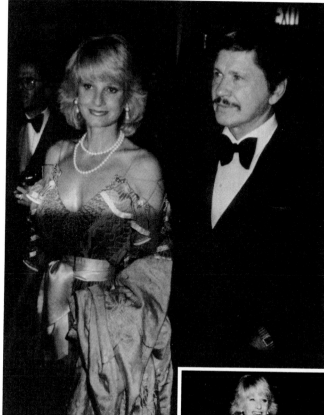

*Two weeks after a fall with
my horse, Stutz, Charles
and I attend a charity dinner,
1983.* (Alan Berliner)

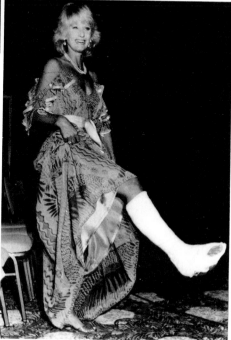

The result of that fall!
(Alan Berliner)

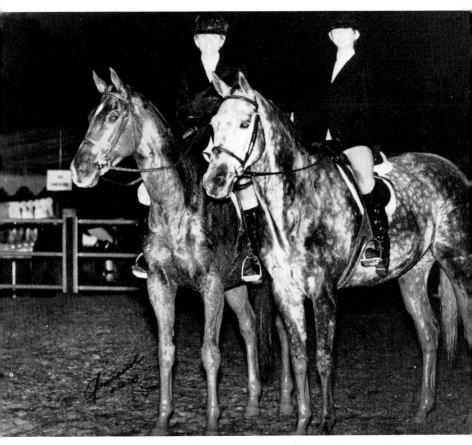

I am on K-Doc and Zuleika is on Robbie, and we are both showing in a rainstorm in Santa Barbara, California, 1983. (Glenncarol Photos)

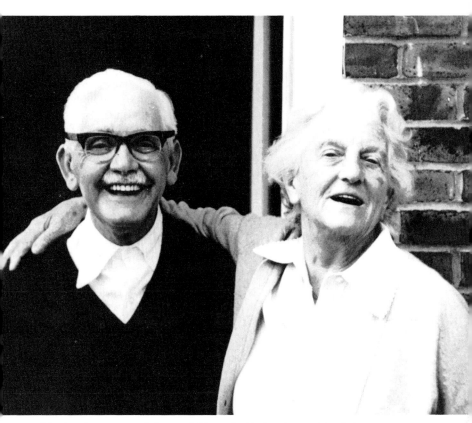

My lovely parents, John and Dorothy Ireland, outside their kitchen door in Seaford, England.

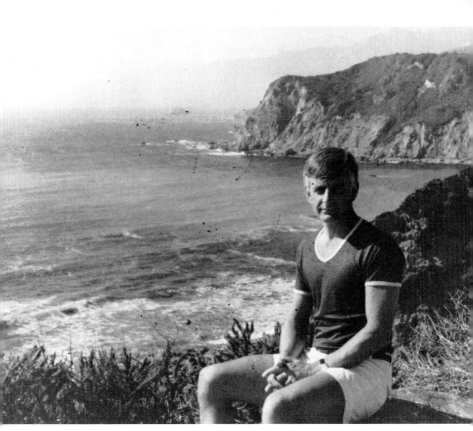

My brother, John Ireland, in Malibu, 1984.

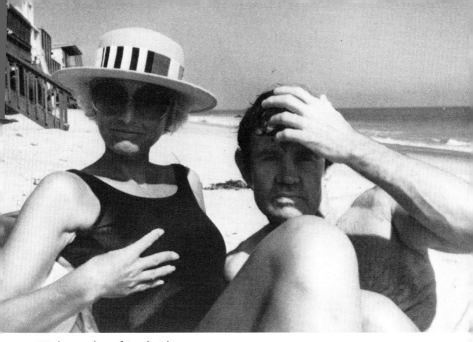

With my dear friend Alan Marshall, also in Malibu, the summer of 1984 after surgery.

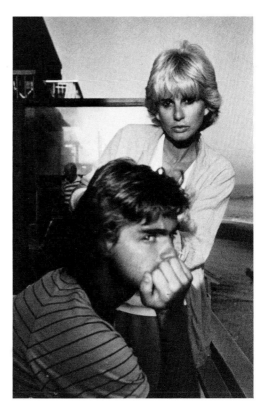

With my son Valentine, that same summer.

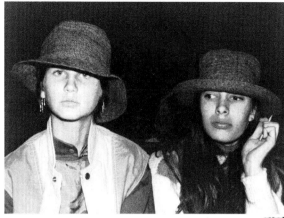

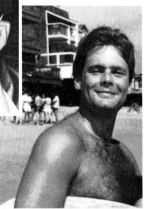

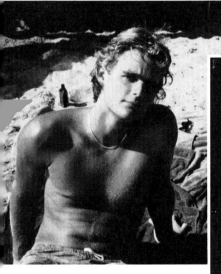

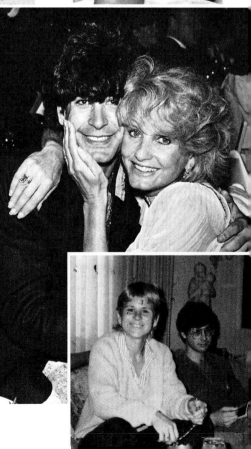

*The children today. Clock-
wise from top left: Zuleika
and Katrina, Paul, Jason
with me at my fiftieth
birthday party,* (Peter C.
Borsari), *Suzanne and
Tony, Valentine.*

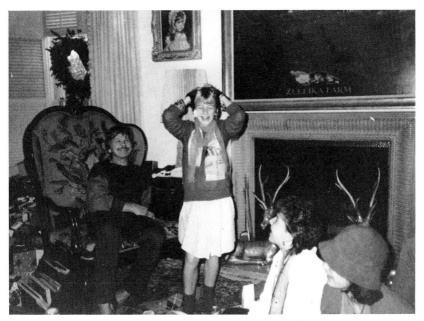

Charles, Courtney, Lindsay and Katrina at our Bel Air house,
celebrating Christmas, 1984.

Here I am with fat cheeks blown up from the last chemotherapy
and glad to be home for Christmas, 1984.

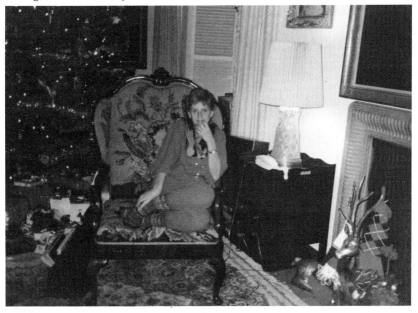

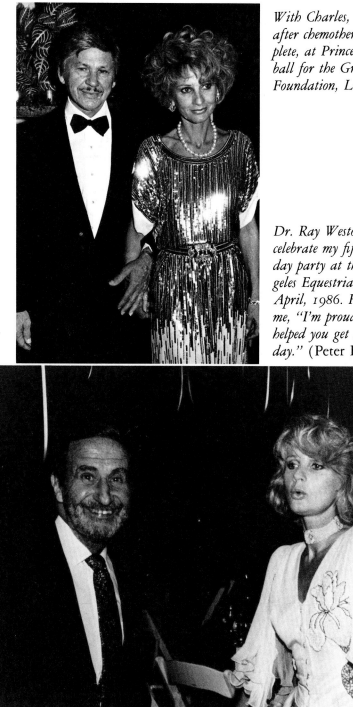

With Charles, seven months after chemotherapy is complete, at Prince Rainier's ball for the Grace Kelly Foundation, Los Angeles.

Dr. Ray Weston helping me celebrate my fiftieth birthday party at the Los Angeles Equestrian Center, April, 1986. He said to me, "I'm proud for having helped you get to this birthday." (Peter Borsari)

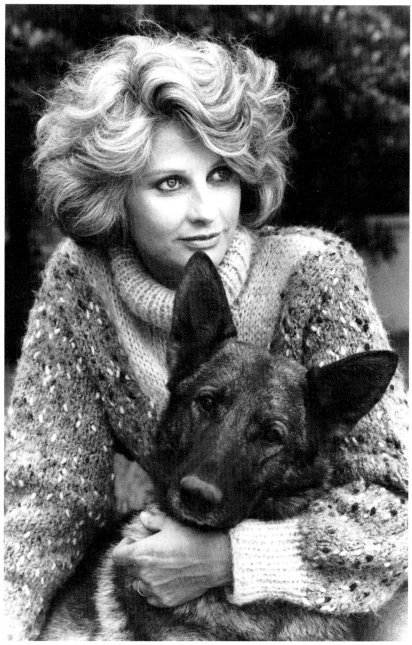

Here I am today, with Cassie. (Charles Bush)

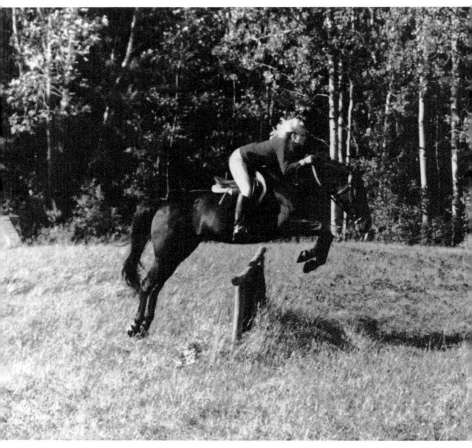

Jumping a fence at Zuleika Farm in Vermont with Psyche. This picture seems to say "Life Wish." (Bridge Hill Studio)

that I should sit in a Jacuzzi or apply hot, wet towels to the area. Mitch told me to call the next day and to come in on Friday if the phlebitis wasn't gone.

It was Valentine's twenty-first birthday. He came to the house for lunch with Paul and I gave him a Rolex watch. "Ooh, that's a mongo watch, Mom, that's really great." I took immense pleasure in the company of Valentine the Great — Valentine the Six-Foot-Seven-Inch Great.

Sometimes, especially when I was with Val, I felt like the incredible shrinking woman. Everyone around me was becoming taller and bigger all the time, while I seemed to be getting smaller, but a little voice said to me, "Not inside, you're not." I knew this to be true. I *was* growing. If I had the courage to keep peeling away layers between myself and my true feelings, my self-knowledge, I knew I would continue to grow and learn. Since infancy, scarcely a year had gone by when I didn't suffer a traumatic physical event. The injuries and illnesses became progressively worse, until finally I hit the jackpot — cancer. Maybe that little baby, isolated in the glass case, thought this was supposed to happen, that she was destined to be ill. I always received admiration and approval for the way I handled my physical calamities. It was something I did well: I made wonderful recoveries. But not anymore. I didn't want it to be necessary to recover anymore. I wanted to get well and stay well. I wanted to reach a point where I didn't need my cancer.

23

THE BIG HOUSE IN BEL AIR resented my absence. Like a monstrous child, it began clamoring for attention. I wouldn't be inside the door more than five minutes before becoming a nervous wreck. My possessions screamed at me: *Take care of us. The staff isn't keeping me bright enough,* shrieked the silver. *There's dust on me,* boomed the grandfather clock and grand piano. *I need polish,* yelled the floors. The windows needed opening. *We need airing,* shouted the twelve bedrooms in unison. *Someone better look at my oven,* called the kitchen.

When I entered the house, the staff waited to hear what I had to say, waited to tell me their problems with running the house in my absence. I visited the dogs. My little collie, Friday, who had been sent to the Bowser Boutique to be dipped and clipped, returned dipped and poodle-clipped, giving him a clownish appearance. The tip of his tail was adorned with a poodle puff. I told Friday he was a fine fellow, and I liked his new summer look, but he wasn't sure. Now, to add insult to injury, there were fleas in his coat.

My beautiful Celia, whom I had brought back from the beach white, fluffy and clean, was now dirty. She too crawled with fleas. It seemed nobody cared for my creatures and things the way I did. There were simply too many things. Every time I visited the house I realized how important it was to change my life-style. Material possessions are a dreadful responsibility.

Sometimes I wished the house would burn down with everything in it, with the exception, of course, of my pets.

I longed for a simpler way of life. I longed for privacy. Maybe I could arrange to have an apartment within all those rooms. Well, why not want "more"? Why not have a small house instead of trying for a small apartment within the big house. I had too many clothes, too many ornaments, too many cups and saucers, sheets, shoes, bags, dogs, horses, children, staff, houses. They were beginning to possess me. Well, no more. I was going to simplify.

I began to believe all my petty illnesses were related to expectations. If I believed something would happen, then it most likely would. To add to the phlebitis in my right arm, I developed phlebitis in my left arm, caused by the chemotherapy needle. Mitchell Karlan gave me an anti-inflammation pill and told me to rest. Rest, rest, rest. Damn rest! I had had it with rest. I felt as if I were in a holding pattern, waiting for my life to begin. I had to work on changing my life patterns. I had to believe I could achieve goals without becoming ill, to believe I could expect to live a normal, healthy life.

Two books rested on my bedside table: O. Carl Simonton's *Getting Well Again* and *Healing from Within* by Dennis T. Jaffe. The books were always within reach. They said the same thing in different ways — that stress and depression made you ill, and your mind could make you well. Cancer occurs when the immune system, white blood cells, ceases to function properly and stops fighting cancer cells. We only have a certain amount of energy in a lifetime and we get into trouble when we use it up too quickly. When that happens, our bodies can no longer resist even the mildest stress. At that point, our energy used up, we break down. I learned that reaction to stress is partly determined by heredity. It's also a response learned from parents or other influential people. I thought of my father's many illnesses.

I read, for instance, that there are men and women who react to stress by tightening the stomach muscles and breathing shallowly as a means of inhibiting emotional reaction. Years later they may find themselves afflicted with lung disease (emphysema), especially if they have irritated the lungs by smoking. Then there are people who express their feelings by inflaming their stomach linings, increasing the risk of ulcers and colitis. My father again sprang to mind. Other people react to emotional or psychological aspects of stress as fighters, blowing out all their emotional energy at once. (Good old Charlie, keep on blowing it out!) That is their form of resistance or stress release. Others do not allow themselves to express the emotional effects of stress and instead localize it in a part of their bodies where it surfaces as headaches, backaches, indigestion or other illnesses. Still others respond to stress with worry, anxiety, depression or chronic tension. I recognized myself in this group.

Completely drained of all energy, the body ceases to defend itself. The results: exhaustion. I remembered the months before my surgery; no matter what I did, exhaustion and fatigue were my constant companions. I had to learn new ways to deal with stress. Obviously, I couldn't be protected from the bumps and bruises of everyday living, but I could learn to deal with life differently, by living in the moment and putting aside a certain amount of time each day to meditate and be alone.

Easier said than done. When I became agitated about all the things I thought I had to do, it was difficult to say, "Now wait a minute. Whoa there, girl, just live in the moment. Do what you have to do right now and don't think of the future." It was difficult to meditate when my brain was overstimulated and anxious. But I would find a way.

One day I returned to the beach house from a visit to the Bel Air house. I was desperate, wondering how I was going to meet the demands of my life. Believe it or not, the deal was back on for the purchase of the House That Jack Built. I knew the house would involve overwhelming work. Renovating would be fun, but moving out of the rented beach house to Bel Air, and then moving to the House That Jack

Built, would not. I was the one who made the plans, who told everyone the way things would be done in these situations. At this point in my recovery, I didn't much fancy the job. Well, I didn't have to do it all right now; I didn't have to plan or think about the future. I only had to stay in the moment. When the time came for me to accept those responsibilities, I would take them one at a time, try not to become overwhelmed nor, more importantly, overstressed.

With those thoughts in mind, I took a walk on the beach with Cassie until I settled down and became conscious of the blue sky, the sea and the sand beneath my toes. Cassie always seemed to mirror my feelings. She would look into my face anxiously and, when I was troubled, she would stay by my side looking up at me. As I relaxed and became more at ease, she became more carefree and ran ahead, bringing sticks and stones for me to throw. I looked for things to pick up, gifts to me from the ocean. I found a wonderful gull's feather, very long and strong. I also found a white, clear stone in the shape of a tear. A teardrop and a feather. I took my gifts back to the house.

When I came in, Charlie groaned. "Jill, I've told you time and time again, stop picking up feathers. They've probably got mites on them."

I just smiled. "They're my gifts from the ocean."

"Not the feathers, Jill. They have mites." I didn't heed him. I washed off my feather and put it in a small vase with the rest of my feather collection. I didn't think they had mites. It wasn't my belief, so they probably didn't, at least not for me.

I had decided to change my theatrical agent. The man who had represented me for a year was a dear person but, unfortunately, was having personal problems at the time. I made an appointment to meet with another agent. I wanted to look good, so Alan made up my face for the first time in seventeen years. I was a little apprehensive. I sat down in the bright sunlight by a window and didn't look until he had finished. He did a beautiful job. I looked really good, not too made up.

Just the eyes were accentuated and a slight base evened out my skin tones. We had thought perhaps I would wear my wig, but it made me uncomfortable.

"This is the way I look, Alan. I think it's more honest to go with my short hair. I feel more myself." I dressed in a peach cotton jumpsuit, combed my short hair and took off for the meeting.

The agent was thirty-six and dynamic. We drank coffee and talked. He was full of energy and constantly interrupted, a person who weaves and searches during a conversation for a handle to express himself and to better understand the other person. He danced with me verbally until we established a rhythm with which we were both comfortable. He asked why I hadn't been doing more work. I told him I had made choices to spend my time with my husband and family.

I told him that when I married Charlie I had had to put my priorities in order. I couldn't travel and work in one part of the world while he worked in another. My choice was to stay with Charlie and keep the children together. I've never regretted it. He said, "I think you were right." He asked if I would like to be represented by his agency.

I said, "Yes, but there's something I should tell you."

"Oh, what's that?"

"I've been ill. I have cancer, but I'm getting better, and, as you can see, I look and feel good."

Well, his mouth fell open. I proceeded to explain that I was comfortable with the fact that I had cancer and I was determined that he should be. I told him I was using a holistic healing approach to make myself well. By the time I'd finished, he told me his brother had cancer and I found myself on a verbal crusade to get him to convince his brother to try holistic healing.

It was an interesting meeting, and I'm sure different from most he held with actresses. When I left the building, I had a new agent and he had a new client, albeit one with cancer. It was good to have Alan make up my face, to dress up and do something like my old self, Jill Ireland, the actress. It must have been mind over matter, because even my hair looked thicker today. It was still very short but — could it be? — there was new hair growing in the bald spots. It was lying on my head in a much more flattering way. Now I just looked as if I had a very, very short haircut. But with my face professionally made up and my eyes accentuated, it was not unflattering. Yea, me! Yea, Alan! Yea, yea, everybody. Now if I could just lose my damned phlebitis, maybe I'd be getting somewhere.

My new agent asked for photographs and a biography. I didn't have a biography, so Alan and his friend Jimmy (with whom Alan lived) listed all the movies and plays I had done in my life. Jimmy typed it up, and Alan took it, along with some photographs I had had taken shortly before my illness, to my agent's office.

I hadn't looked at the photographs since before my surgery, and what I saw then were pictures of a glamorous, sophisticated woman wearing evening gowns, at least the top half of evening gowns. The camera didn't show the bottom half of Jill clad in blue jeans with one leg of the material cut away to reveal a removable cast with metal braces. The pictures were beautifully lighted. I was exquisitely made up and coiffed, the portraits had been artfully retouched and the finished product was gorgeous. I studied the photographs now with a cold, analytical eye. I knew it was me — I remembered very clearly the day of the sitting — but I felt greatly removed and different from the woman with the broken leg that refused to heal. I thought I knew something about patience that day, but I knew much more about it now.

24

BETWEEN MY FIFTH AND SIXTH chemotherapy treatments I found a delightful and slightly off-beat diversion that lightened the heavy cloud under which I found myself much of the time. *Astrology.*

I hadn't seen an astrologer for twenty years. Chakrapani was highly recommended and different from other astrologers. He was very skilled, said to be one of India's greatest, with thirty years of practice in his ancient art. Chakrapani based his readings on the Vedic system. His readings were said to be cosmic in depth and psychic in nature. A friend made the appointment for me, giving only the date, time and place of my birth. I looked forward to a little light entertainment.

Chakrapani was a friendly, jolly little man who seemed to enjoy doing my chart, at least we laughed a lot. At first, I found it hard to understand Chakrapani. He spoke in a funny singsong voice, mixing an Indian accent with what sounded like New York Yiddish expressions, which made me want to giggle. I was still English enough to suppress it, but only just. He sounded like Peter Sellers doing an Indian. Alan had accompanied me, and I wondered if he was thinking the same thing. I didn't dare meet his eyes, afraid he'd make me laugh.

Chakrapani shuffled my chart on the desk, shifted in his seat and looked at me searchingly. Then he settled back, closed his eyes and began in his singsong voice:

"This chart has tremendous power. There is a lot of energy

in this chart. You are a woman of depth. There is tremendous dimension in your personality. You are a very strong person, even though your mind is twenty-five hours busy in a twenty-four-hour day. Do you understand? That means it is over-busy."

Alan broke out laughing. He was losing control and I was about to join him. I flashed him a look. Quiet, Alan!

"Overbusy?"

"It is twenty-five hours busy in a twenty-four-hour day. What does it mean? It is too busy. You are a woman who has faced life, challenges of life, like nobody's business. Is it not true?"

Alan was nodding his head up and down like an old Chinese mandarin. Oh, yes, oh, yes, he punctuated his nods.

"You have seen ups and downs like nobody's business. You have gone through life like nobody's business. You don't want to even look at it, how you've gone through. I would say you've gone through — experienced — miracles in the course of your life, because at some times in your life you have thought you were finished and nobody can save you. You are gone for good. Did you not think like that? Yes. Well, some-how, as the time passed, you are saved and protected."

I sat perfectly still on the stiff, little straight-backed chair. I didn't know what to think. I said little. I was determined not to give anything away. I wanted it all to come from him. Alan was having a fine time, however, laughing and nodding agreement at what was being said.

"That is the power of Guru. Guru is the power of protection. It is always behind you. Even though in 1984 you have experienced troubles and problems and tension and anxiety and difficulty and problems, and problems like nobody's business in 1985 also, there is no doubt."

He sang through that little speech with the virtuosity of an auctioneer. The rapidity of his speech astounded me.

"Nineteen eighty-four is one of the most strugglesome years you have experienced in recent years. That is why June, July, August were very difficult months. Whole year — you know — but they are the climaxes. It is getting finished."

I suddenly became very interested. "Even healthwise? Health is very important to me right now."

He nodded sagely.

"In everything. Anything that is connected with that. Everything is getting finished in the same way."

Oh, God, I hoped he was right.

With another quick look at my charts, Chakrapani continued:

"Very good. Now your rising sign is occupied by Guru. Guru is called the planet of knowledge and wisdom and learning and study and growth and progress and prosperity and dignity."

Off he went again in his rapid chant. Only now, I had no desire to laugh. He was singing my life. I was hooked.

"A woman of dignity. You carry a certain amount of personal dignity wherever you go. Rahu has also given you some health complaints in the form of skin rashes, allergies and a cut, a wound, an operation."

Whoa, boy! At this, I rocked back and really paid attention.

"It gives you even that. And it began strongly sometime from January 1982 onwards. Slowly it began to catch up with you."

Uh-huh. Truly captivated, I was scarcely breathing.

"And '83 and '84 you experienced . . . you are connected with doctors and medicine and health like nobody's business, especially January, February, March, April, May, June, July, August 1984. That's the power of this Rahu. Rahu is concerned with your health."

I couldn't believe my ears. He was really on a roll. I said, "I hope it's finished. I hope the illnesses are finished."

"I think it is finished, but you still have to be careful. What you have to be careful about is your body is very hot."

Very hot. I was shocked. Nobody knew about the hot, burning sensations since the chemotherapy.

"Inside the body is hot. The moment the body is hot, you are due for trouble. The body becomes hot by too much

162

thinking, worry, tension, not enough sleep. That is why you should eat a lot of cooling food, not a lot of meat. Meat is not good for that, because it creates too much heat in the body. Why don't you eat some steamed vegetables and a lot of water you should drink — a lot. Yes, it is good for you, because this will keep your body system cool."

"I've had a lot of illness," I said.

"He'll tell *you*," said Alan.

"It has been from '65 onwards your health complaints have begun to grow. In '54 and '55 also, you had some problems of health. So it is going back. When you were a child, your health problem is there. But you have got a strong health. I want to tell you that also. You have tremendously strong health. And you have got health problems. Both are true. Your body is strong. It can withstand pressures. It can withstand anything. It's like steel. It means even if you get a cut, wound, operation, it gets healed. That's what I mean. It has the power of healing. And power to suffer, and suffering is there, of course. Both are there."

He took a short pause, then smiled sweetly at me.

"You are a woman of opposites, a woman of contradictions, an unconventional revolutionary. You are a person who has a great sense of justice and fairness and truth and righteousness. All this is true. At the same time, you want it exactly the way you want it. You'll listen to no one."

"Oh, you're so right, Chakrapani. She *won't*," Alan interrupted.

"Be quiet, Alan, this is my dime."

Chakrapani rustled through the papers in front of him.

"In '86, '87 '88, you will make some progress."

"I'm glad to hear I'll be around in '86, '87, '88."

"You've got a long life. Didn't I tell you you had a body of steel?"

"I hope so."

"Didn't I tell you that?"

"Yes, you did. So you see I have a long life? You can see that?"

"Of course."

"This means a great deal to me at this period of my life."

"Yes, you've got a long life. There is no doubt about it."

"I have cancer . . ."

"It doesn't matter."

"And I've had surgery . . ."

"Doesn't matter."

"But I feel strong, inside me."

"You're bound to be strong."

"Oh, that's good. You project a long life for me?"

"Yes, definitely. You have physically suffered. That's okay."

I agreed. "I don't mind that, but I want something to come of my suffering. I don't mind suffering if it's not just thrown to the wind; if out of it comes something I can build with."

Alan touched me gently. "Oh, but it's coming, Jill. It's happening."

"You have tremendous willpower. Whatever you accept you are able to hold on to by your will. It's a life force."

He continued, boogidy, boogidy, boogidy, through my chart.

"I tell you, your luck is going to improve on February, March, April, May 1985. Something is going to change that will bring happiness."

I was glowing.

"Of course, more than one marriage is indicated."

Whoops! "How many?"

"I don't know."

"You don't know? Well, give me a ballpark figure." We all laughed. Then I began to feel a little uncomfortable. "By marriages, do you mean legal marriages or just associations?"

"Legal."

"Legal marriages. More than one is indicated?"

"Yes."

"Well, that's all right so far." I pushed it. "Is it more than two?"

This brought more laughter from all three of us. But

Chakrapani wasn't disposed to discuss my marital situations any further. He dismissed further questioning by closing his eyes, placing his fingertips together and leaning back in his chair. There was a small silence while he seemed to think hard. Suddenly, he looked at me almost with a question.

"Twelfth house. How is your leg? Do you have experience with pain in the leg?"

This was getting too close for comfort. "I broke my leg and the bone wouldn't heal. Sometimes it still gives me pain."

"Yes, that's what it is."

"I have injured my leg four times."

"You should take care of that. It is Saturn's aspect on Sun in Mars and Mercury. It creates problems in the leg."

"For all my life?"

"Yes, you should be always watchful for that. Never take risks."

"Do you think I should stop riding and jumping horses?"

"Totally."

My hear sank. "Totally? You think I should? Are you sure?"

"Yes."

"I love riding. I'm very reluctant to give it up."

"Well, you want to suffer, you should do it."

"No, I don't want to suffer, but I like to ride my horses. You really see that I should give up riding?"

"Yes. You see these problems — it will create more problems after for your leg."

"How about running?"

"No good. Swimming. Why don't you swim?"

"I'm a lousy swimmer. It hurts my ears."

"Why should it hurt your ears?"

"Because if the water goes in my ears . . ."

"You plug the ears."

"And I have to get wet."

"Plug the ears. You can get wet."

"No. I don't like getting myself wet."

Chakrapani looked at me for a moment, then, realizing I was being facetious, he relaxed, leaned back in his chair and laughed uproariously.

I felt rather depressed, but I said, "I'm going to listen to what you said about the legs and the risk. Don't take risks." I said it, but deep down in my heart I knew nothing would make me give up my horses and riding them.

"Your Saturn cycle has begun. It will uplift you like nobody's business. Nineteen eighty-three was the beginning of the benefits of the Saturn coming to you. Even though you have suffered in 1984, it has nothing to do with Saturn. Saturn only brought it up to be removed. It has been there before. It has been there from 1975 onwards. Slowly you are building up. Because of emotions and frustrations and tensions — '75, '76, '77, '78, '79, '80, '81, '82 — including '82. The suppression of emotions brought this kind of a problem to you. It's the emotional suppression."

Bonk! It seemed to me I'd heard this song before. He began to sound very much like an Indian Dr. Simonton.

"You controlled many things, without reasoning out by understanding. Control is not good, but understanding is good. Does it make sense to you?"

It had all begun to sound very familiar. Sue Colin couldn't have put it better. I was reminded of words from the song "How Long Has This Been Going On?": "I could cry icy tears, where have I been all these years?" I was getting the same message from everyone. It all seemed so clear to me now. How could I have been so slow to understand these things that everybody else seemed to know so well?

He consulted my chart again, muttering to himself under his breath.

"As your health problems come, your luck will begin to grow."

"As they come, my luck will grow?"

"Yes, it has some connection. Ninth house ruler situated in the fifth house brought some obstructions and difficulties in the area of children. How is that? Obstruction and obstacles

166

in relation to children. Abortion, miscarriage, problems in delivery. Health problems with the children you have borne?"

I had to agree. Problems of delivery and miscarriage were things that had happened. I was amazed. How could he read all this in my chart? He went on.

"And if the children are born, health problems for the children?"

"No, not so far." (I had forgotten for the moment about Paul's kidney stone.)

"Not so far? Okay, good."

I couldn't believe I was sitting in this strange man's house listening to what I knew Charlie would call gypsy fortune-telling. Chakrapani seemed to be just plucking my life out of the air. Even Alan didn't know about my miscarriages. Now he began to refer to what I recognized as my hopes for a new house.

"You will have luck with property that is going to come to you."

"Property?" (Oh, this was good news.)

"Yes."

"You mean like . . ."

"Land. Building. Yes. Luck in that is indicated. And you will have one of the most beautiful houses. You will have it."

"That's good."

Chakrapani settled in for another gallop down the track.

"Health complaints, disputes and conflicts and struggle."

I wanted to stop him. Enough already with the struggles and conflicts.

"But somehow you're always protected by Guru's aspect. That is why I tell you to take care of your leg."

Oh, no, not my leg again. Please!

"*Do not* take risks there. You are passing through the Saturn cycle, and the major cycle of Saturn operates until April 1986. By April 1986, your life takes root. Yes. 'Eighty-seven is going to be one of the best years you will be experiencing."

"Good. Whew! It's about time after all those struggles, conflicts and disputes."

"Yes, '87. Still that means till '86 there is some struggle you will experience. I don't want to give you false promise. Okay? It is there until 1986. Hopefully, it will end then."

"Do you see health problems through '85?"

"Concern. I don't say problem, I say concern. Feeling limited. That means I want you to take caution, that's all, in what you eat and what you do. Don't take physical risks."

"I'll have to stop jumping my horses then."

"You should jump from the second floor of the building."

Everyone laughed. Mister Chakrapani was a bit of a smart ass.

"No jumping, I would say, at least," Alan joined in smugly.

Well, they'd pretty much immobilized me. I was suddenly tired but there were still more questions I wanted to ask. I wanted it all — complete reassurance, a stamp of approval, all hopes returned.

"Chakrapani, my biggest concern is the length of time I am going to live. With cancer, you know, you live under . . . I'm strong, like you say, but every now and then when something happens, you think, oh, God, maybe I'm really fooling myself. Maybe I'm not as strong . . ."

"I know people who live twenty-five years," he said quietly.

"Oh, I'm planning a long life but, at the same time, you do have fears. And the statistics are all against you." (My vulnerability was showing. I was going to buy whatever he said.)

"No fear. No fear for your life. I told you, you have a health problem, but you have a body of steel."

"I've always been accident-prone. I've had accidents all my life."

"But still you survive it. You are physically strong. You look here and now physically strong."

"I have a phlebitis problem today." God, next I would tell him I'd lost my pubic hair.

"It is bound to be that way with stress."

"Due to stress? Physical stress?"

"Mental stress. You have gone through a lot of mental stress."

Alan, seeing my anxiety, put a stop to all this. "Listen, one more time, to your life expectancy. Is she going to live to be an old woman?"

"Yes."

"Now is that enough? He sees you as an old woman. Are you happy now? You're going to be an old, old hag. Satisfied?" Everyone laughed but I still wanted more. I wanted it all back, all my innocence, all my future.

"But I don't want to be an old, ill woman. I want to be an old, vital, strong . . ."

"Yes, yes. You will always be moving around."

"You don't see me on crutches?"

"No."

"But I see her as a nagging old woman." Alan had had it. He was hungry and ready for lunch. Piss off, Alan.

"But you don't see me as an old . . . I would fear very much being an old, helpless woman. I want to be strong."

"You will never live as a helpless woman."

"Never?"

"Never."

"Oh, good. Thank you very much."

Chakrapani thanked me as I paid him, and he saw us to the door. It had been worth every penny of the one hundred dollars I'd given him. I'd just bought myself a long, healthy life, cheap at the price.

25

CHAKRAPANI'S READING GAVE ME much on which to dwell. The part about not riding horses and the warning about my legs got to me. I wasn't riding at the moment because of the phlebitis in both arms. Mitchell Karlan told me I shouldn't drive or take long walks or do anything else strenuous until the phlebitis disappeared.

Alan turned up on Thursday morning to drive me to my appointments. The first was with Michael, my oncologist, for a blood test. It went smoothly enough. The second was with my surgeon or, more accurately, his associate, Dr. Uyeda. Mitch was out of town.

Alan was excited. He had made an appointment for me with a very fine plastic surgeon who, Alan assured me, would create a pair of perfect breasts — "like centerpieces." He was keen that I should have the surgery before Christmas. I said it was too soon, but I went along with Alan's enthusiasm. By the time we arrived at the doctor's office, he had almost convinced me to have my breasts done and have the tip of my nose shortened as well. In fact, the way Alan saw it, I was going to be in better shape than before the cancer.

Earlier, we visited Bernard Dowson, who was back in business. The difference was semantics. To all intents, he was going to teach me meditation. He said he hoped to be in business for the next forty years and that he had to protect himself. I was glad to see him again under any circumstances. Bernard made me feel better.

Alan and I took the table treatment, so we were both in a fine mood. And it was with a feeling of well-being that I waited for Robert Uyeda to tell me how soon I could have the reconstructive surgery. Dr. Uyeda looked at me and then kindly but firmly told me I should wait at least a year after completing my chemotherapy. He said complete healing wouldn't take place until then. Also, the stage of my cancer must be taken into account in determining whether I could *ever* have reconstructive surgery. In some cases, it wasn't advisable. He said if there was a recurrence, it usually took place within the first or second year. Therefore, it would be better to wait, because reconstructive surgery made it more difficult to detect cancer in the early stages.

I brought Alan in from the waiting room and had Dr. Uyeda repeat what he'd told me. Alan was stunned and disappointed. Dr. Uyeda reiterated, "Consideration must be given the stage of the tumor when surgery is done, and in some cases surgery is not advisable."

Back in the car, Alan was beside himself. Furious. "Well," he said, "I have no faith in the AMA. Your doctor is very nice and I respect him and what he said, but my faith is in holistic healing."

I was somewhat unnerved. The phrase "stage of the tumor" sounded ominous. I found myself sinking into a bit of depression, as concerned about Alan as I was by Dr. Uyeda's words. Alan cared so much and I didn't want him to feel I was disappointed about reconstructive surgery. He had trouble handling the whole thing. I pointed out that I had to be realistic, that recurrence was possible and maybe I could lose my left breast.

There was no way Alan would listen to such a suggestion. He kept repeating, "No, I won't hear it. You're not going to have a recurrence, and I don't like to think of you living with a sword over your head."

"I'm not living with a sword over my head, Alan. The sword is there, but it's not hanging over my head. It's way off to the right in the corner. It's there — I acknowledge that — but not hanging over my head. I'm not worried, so please don't be upset."

We drove home to find the beach house empty and I didn't have a key. Charlie had gone to watch Zuleika compete in a swim meet for her school. Alan scaled the wall and let us in. We were depressed and uneasy, so Alan had a glass of wine and a cigarette while I took a walk on the beach with Cassie until I felt more like myself.

I kept hearing the doctor's words: "stage of the tumor," "inadvisable in some cases," "maybe in Jill's case it is not advisable," "recurrences usually happen within the first one or two years." Cassie charged ahead to chase birds. I wished I could run with her. I would like to have dashed ahead and left all my thoughts and feelings behind. Strangely enough, I wasn't really depressed or frightened. It was simply a bit of a downer.

For the past few days, even with the phlebitis, I had felt better knowing I had no more cancer. But now, of course, I knew I would have to wait out the next two years. There would be moments of anxiety and fear to face for sure. Well, nobody said it would be easy. After twenty minutes on the beach, I turned my back to the sun and walked to the house. Now I was feeling better. The sea had done what it always did; it had relaxed me.

I found, as expected, Alan had gone home, leaving a message he would call later. He was so involved with me and my illness; he wanted so much for me to be better and perfect that these little setbacks were hard on him. Things weren't going well in his own life and I thought perhaps he chose to worry about me rather than himself. I felt I was disappointing him. I wanted to be well for such a good friend, a lifeline. I was in no hurry to have the breast transplant done, but I would have liked to do it for Alan. His vision of me all put together and lovely was much too tempting to resist.

I had to return to square one. Maybe we were becoming too cocky, Alan and I, about my complete recovery. I should go back and start one more time. Start meditating three times a day. I had let it slip to once a day. And get back to my diet. I had let that slip, too. The job wasn't over. The road was longer and, so far, relief was not in sight. I was reminded of these lines, "The woods are lovely, dark and deep. But I have promises to keep."

It was mid-October, three days before chemotherapy six. I resolved to be a good girl until then, but, perversely, even as I determined to return to my regimen, I found myself hunting through the house for chocolate that I knew I had hidden some time ago. I made myself a cup of tea. "Feeling a little down, dear? Have a cup of tea." With my tea and chocolate, I crept into a little spare bedroom that I used for meditation and writing, all the while feeling guilty and furtive. The chocolate didn't taste that good, but I ate it nevertheless.

I hadn't realized how much I had counted on reconstructive surgery. It hadn't meant anything until I was told it wasn't advisable in some cases. While the option was open to me, I could be independent and not want to have it, but should that option be closed, how would I feel? I needed Charlie. I wanted to talk to him. I sat cross-legged on the floor with my back to the wall in a corner and meditated. But Charlie's little pig couldn't concentrate. My mind wandered to earlier in the day when Alan and I were rattling along in beat-up old Granny with Cassie looking balefully carsick in the backseat.

I had asked him, "Alan, do you think I'll ever work again as an actress, now that I'm incomplete in a manner of speaking?"

"Of course you will, darling, but you have to have a great part and a wonderful director. It should be a woman or maybe somebody gay."

"Great," I said. "I'll advertise in the trade papers: *One-titted actress seeks employment from a faggot director who'll understand.*"

"But you won't be one-titted, cookie. We're going to have

you reconstructed. They're going to be beautiful — center-pieces."

Oh, well, back to the grindstone. I closed my eyes and once again tried to meditate. This time I was more successful. I seemed to have laid to rest most of the things that were whirling in my brain, what author Dennis Jaffe called "roof brain chatter." I loved that expression. Roof brain chatter. It so accurately described what went on in my head most of the time, an unending conversation with myself. My meditation went quite well. My white blood cells competently coursed around my body doing their job, hunting down and destroying cancer cells as they found them. When I finished with that portion of my meditation, I worked on my convictions.

I thought back to Chakrapani's astrological findings, how he said mine was a very powerful chart. I worked on the feeling of power. He said I had a body of steel. I worked on that. I visualized myself with a body of steel. I thought of all the positive and strong things he had said to reinforce my belief that I would be well and have a long, healthy life. If I allowed myself to believe I would have a cancer recurrence within the next year or two, then I probably would. But if I deeply believed I would not — that my white cells would take care of all stray cancer cells in my system at this moment — then I knew I wouldn't suffer a recurrence. Too bad it wasn't that easy. It takes enormous work to change one's beliefs. Dr. Simonton knew that when he had me meditate and think positive, strong images of health and power and make a fist to reinforce these good, healthful convictions.

Using that method, I began thinking of myself with a body of steel, able to withstand many things. Whenever I felt insecure or out of control, I would simply make a fist to bring forth the positive feelings associated with that gesture. Once again, I realized an illness like cancer could not be dealt with totally by the American Medical Association. Spiritually, one had to heal and grow to deal with the future as well as the present.

However, I also realized part of my depression this particular day was the shock of coming up against the reality of my disease in the eyes of the AMA. Dr. Uyeda had told me, "We know very little about cancer and how to treat it in 1984. We cut out the tumor and all the surrounding tissue. We treat it with a cannon. It's the best we can do right now."

It really was incredibly crude, I thought, cutting slices off the body that way. How important to keep in contact with one's white blood cells, keep them working, *never* let them slack off. The mind is very powerful; we have only to harness it and make it work for us and do what we want it to do. I believed that in this particular field, anything goes — anything that will help the patient come into his own power. My mind had been thrashing around for several months, but it was beginning to settle down.

The day after my visit to Dr. Uyeda, Charlie and I faced the fact that negotiations for our house were not going our way. I had hoped to be in escrow and perhaps working on the house by Christmas. But we were no further advanced than we had been three months earlier. Every time we were prepared to close the deal, with pen in the air, ready to sign, the sellers came up with another clause totally unacceptable to us. I wanted the house so desperately I had put Charlie in a difficult position. He had no power to negotiate. The owners knew how much I coveted the place. They also knew I was ill and the word was out that Charles Bronson would buy his wife anything she wanted.

I called our broker and said, "Madeline, I've had it. I want you to call the Skinners and tell them to please put their house back on the market. I'm taking my marbles and going home."

She couldn't believe it. "But, Jill, the house is perfect for you."

"It *was* perfect for me, Madeline, three months ago. But they've given us too much time to think and now I want you to tell them to eat it — raw."

She was shocked. "You mean you don't want the house? You really mean it?"

"I mean I've lost interest in the house. I really mean it." She hung up. My heart pounded. I couldn't believe what I'd done.

Charlie looked at me askance. He couldn't believe it either. "But, Jill, you really want that house."

"I do want it, Charlie, I really do. But I won't let anybody fuck me over anymore, and I won't let them fuck you over either." The phone rang as I voiced my thoughts. It was Madeline's superior at the real estate office — a very cool lady. I repeated my feelings.

She said, "All right." That was *all* she said. Clever woman.

However, before she *could* speak, I said, "We have the necessary down payment and we're going to buy ourselves another house. Tell your clients to put their house on the market again and if, further down the line, we haven't found something else we prefer, we *may* come back to their house *if* they drop the price."

Again, my heart pounded. I felt sick. I couldn't believe I was doing it. What was going on with me? What was going on was that I had taken enough. My basic nature is agreeable. I let people take advantage of me for a long time before I turn around, but when I make up my mind I can be very stubborn. Chakrapani was right. However, I knew I wasn't playing with a light issue here. It was an emotional one. I was talking about our future home, but I felt this inner energy and I wasn't about to let them get the better of me. The telephone rang again. The real estate office was back.

"The Skinners want to know if you would like to have a meeting on Sunday." Charlie had answered the phone this time. I heard his reply.

"On Sunday? I don't know if we can do it Sunday. A meeting? Let me ask my wife." He asked, "Do you want to have a meeting?"

By now I was contrary. Besides, these calls told me there

was a shift in power. "No," I said. "Fuck them. I don't want to have a meeting. Tell them I'm not in the mood."

Charlie told her we weren't interested. As far as we were concerned, the deal was off. He hung up. Oh, my God, I couldn't believe it. What had I done? I grabbed the big real estate book with photographs of other houses and started frantically leafing through it.

"Come and sit down, we have to talk about this," I said to Charlie. "Where shall we live?"

Charlie looked at me long and hard. "How about Oregon?"

I started to laugh. "Well, if you're going to be absurd, we can't talk at all. There's only one thing to do. Let's go upstairs."

"I'm with you," he said, and we spent a wondrous few hours rolling around in bed having a good time.

At dinner that night Alan was in a particularly jolly mood. He and his friend Jimmy joined Charlie and me and Zuleika at a rustic restaurant in Topanga Canyon. Katrina was at ballet class and would stay the night with a friend. Alan told us he had landed a job on a movie with Jill Clayburgh on location on Cape Cod. I wondered in the back of my mind what it would be like without Alan. Since I had been living at the beach, Alan had been there for me whenever I needed him. When I was too ill to drive, he drove me. When I needed cheering, he cheered me. But I was happy for Alan. I knew I would miss him, but I was so much stronger now. Because of him, I was more independent. So it was a celebration dinner. We drank health-food wine and ate health-food food. We hugged each other good-bye, and I told Alan I would see him in a week.

26

THE NEXT DAY I WENT TO the hairdresser to have my legs waxed and my eyelashes dyed. I'd never had my eyelashes dyed and thought it was a splendid plan. I still was troubled by the phlebitis, but I tried not to think about it. The girl who waxed my legs asked about my health. She knew I had cancer, but she didn't know where, so I told her I had had a mastectomy. She was interested. Many people didn't ask questions, but she did. And I sensed she really wanted to know the answers. She asked how I had known I had cancer, and if it hurt. I told her very little pain is involved in breast removal because many nerves are removed, too. In fact, I still had no feeling under my right arm and down my right side almost five months after surgery. I told her anyone facing similar surgery should not be afraid, that it wasn't so bad. She thanked me.

Dyeing my eyelashes was not a great success. It didn't seem to make any difference. I had long lashes, but they were very blond. After the dye job, they still seemed blond. Oh, well, it was fun doing it and I enjoyed talking to the beautician.

People in the little Malibu commercial center, where I shopped, were accustomed to seeing me walk around with my short haircut, followed by Cassie. I felt I was making contacts and a few budding friendships. Everyone I talked with seemed to know we were buying a house on Old Malibu Road. I couldn't believe word had traveled so fast in the community, but it had.

So I changed my story. "Well, we may not be buying it," I told people who asked. "We're having trouble with the negotiations, and we're not in escrow. I'm beginning to look at other houses." I hoped word would get back to the real estate agents and the owners of the House That Jack Built.

The pain in my left arm was troublesome. I called Ray Weston, who told me to apply moist heat. I had stopped taking the pills he gave me after Bernard tested them and told me they were toxic. The upset stomach and headaches I had suffered while taking them stopped immediately. I don't know how much of my reaction was psychosomatic. The way my mind traveled at that time, psychosomatic was just another word for many things that happened to me. I didn't want to become too hypochondriacal, but every little pain bothered me. Not the actual sensation of pain, but *what* I imagined it might be. Oh, boy! I was a typical case — classic. In the extensive reading I'd done, all cancer patients said they imagined every little pain to be cancer, and here I was doing the same thing. But I couldn't ignore pains. What if they were cancer? I lay awake most of the night nursing my bad arm. I worried the phlebitis might forestall chemo six on Monday. Then again, I didn't want a needle sliding into my arm with a vein full of blood clots. The thought troubled me, but I decided I would go for my therapy on Monday anyhow and discuss it with Michael.

The next day I did something new for me. I listened to my body, which told me I was pushing myself. I wasn't feeling well. My arm hurt and I was exhausted. I confessed to Charlie and Zuleika and asked if they would go to the horse show without me. It was a difficult decision. I had looked forward to seeing all my buddies, and I always enjoyed watching Zuleika ride. However, I did what everyone had been telling me to do for the past three months: I stayed home and nurtured myself.

After seeing Zuleika and Charlie off at six in the morning, I went to bed and slept. Awaking at 10:30, I made tea and toast and got back into bed. I called my mother in England and talked for an hour and a half. I didn't bother dressing. I let Cassie out on the beach to play with the Doberwoman next door. I did some reading and meditated, luxuriating in pressureless time to myself. I put a heating pad on my arm and kept it elevated as instructed.

Later, Paul and Priscilla, his girlfriend, stopped by to talk about their forthcoming camping trip. Paul was an avid hiker; Priscilla wasn't so sure. She wondered if they could take a portable shower and toilet to install in the tent. We thought that was funny and told Priscilla she had the wrong idea about camping. She had to give in to her baser nature and allow herself to get a bit grubby.

Katrina came home and listened to the conversation before saying, "Oh, I went on a camping trip once. I didn't go to the bathroom for two days because they wanted me to do it in a ditch."

Priscilla said, "Oh, my God, what did you do?"

"I ate a lot of cheese. I refused to go in their ditch. I wouldn't have minded my own personal ditch, but I had to use theirs and they were watching."

"Well, no wonder you didn't want to go," I said. "I wouldn't want to go with everyone watching."

We tried to teach Priscilla how it was possible to pee standing up. Katrina cautioned her about squatting down and peeing in case of poison ivy or nettle stings. Priscilla grew less and less enthusiastic about the trip. She suggested they stay in a motel and Paul could hike around and around it. Paul said, "No way, you're going on a camping trip."

It was a pleasant afternoon. I enjoyed their company while doing what I wanted and needed — resting. Priscilla was making a model airplane on the veranda, Cassie was asleep on a float and Paul was watching television. I went upstairs to be alone and meditate.

Katrina and Zuleika were fascinated, as had been their

friends Marin and Rachel, when I meditated. They had wanted to join me. So the girls and I would all sit cross-legged on the floor, holding crystals, while I talked them through a meditation, telling them to relax and describing in a soothing voice pleasant scenes for them to visualize. I made tapes for them, and each night after their homework I would hear the sound of my own voice coming out of the girls' rooms.

That night I went in to say good night to Zuleika. She was lying in bed holding a crystal and playing the meditation tape I had made for her. Looking at my daughter, I was very moved. I promised I would make her another meditation tape. She had almost memorized the one to which she was listening.

Before going to bed I drank a bottle of white wine and told Charlie I didn't want to die of cancer. I wasn't depressed. I was almost jolly. I said, "No way do I want to die of cancer."

"If you don't want to, you probably won't."

"You bet I won't. I'll take my car and drive off the end of San Vincente Boulevard and fly onto Pacific Coast Highway first."

"Perhaps you wouldn't die."

"If I knew it was terminal, I'd settle my affairs and that's what I would do." I didn't mean it, at least I didn't think I did, but I said it anyhow.

Chemotherapy number six was due the next day, and I went to bed a little bit drunk.

I woke up at 6:30 Monday morning and took a Decadron, the anti-inflammation drug that always heralded the start of a chemo day. I was to take one every six hours, so I swallowed a tablet as early as possible in order to get another into my system before the chemo. Then I kissed Zuleika awake. I lay beside her and snuggled into the curve of her body. "I love you, darling. Have a good day. I'll see you later."

"I love you, Mom. I'll see you later, too."

I spent the balance of the morning in bed. I simply pulled the covers over my head. I didn't want to speak to anybody.

For some reason, chemotherapy number six was like a

comedy half hour. I could never stand the smell of the ice helmet. It had a distinct rubbery odor, and it always made me feel sick, so when Michelle put the tourniquet on my head, I held a Kleenex over my nose. That made it difficult for Charlie to hold my hand during therapy. So I took two Kleenex and shoved one up each nostril. They actually hung out of my nose like two long strings of mucus. That made Michelle and Charlie laugh so hard tears ran down their faces. In a nasal voice, I said to her sternly, "Michelle, do you always laugh at your patients? Is this the way you carry on in here?"

Her face straightened immediately, and she said, "Oh, no, this is very serious business."

"Then why are you laughing?" She cracked up again. My next question was about reconstructive surgery. She said she'd met a lot of women who'd had it done, and they'd all been pleased. Then I said, "But Michelle, what would happen if I had a breast implant, and then, when I'm sixty, if I live that long, I'll have one youthful, girlish breast and a long, pendulus one."

Again, more hysterical laughter. "Michelle, please take me seriously." I was having a ball, but if she laughed too hard, the needle might waggle in my arm, so I tried to be serious. I asked about a very together patient whom I had seen the week before when I'd had my blood test. The woman came out of her treatment on top of everything. She remarked how we had to keep our hair short for a while and then gave me advice on shampoos and how I should avoid combing or touching my hair whenever I could. I said, "Michelle, that is some lady. I don't come out of my treatments that together. Do you mean to say I'm the only one who snivels, whimpers and whines?"

More laughter. She replied, "You don't whine, Jill."

"How about the sniveling and whimpering?"

"Well, maybe a little." More laughter.

Our laughter had been loud and long. It felt good, but we were a noisy bunch.

I said, "Good Lord, people are going to wonder what's

going on. This really is your once-every-three-weeks comedy hour."

Michael came in. "What's going on in here?"

"It's just Michelle enjoying herself while giving me my treatment." I asked Michael about reconstructive surgery and told him how keen Alan was for me to have it.

"Don't do it for Alan," he said. "Do it for yourself if you must. It's major surgery, and there's always a risk element in surgery. But I will say this, Jill. Every woman I know who has done it is thrilled. It solves so many problems. You can dress normally and you feel renewed and whole again."

This cheered me up. That and Michelle's lusty laughter during my chemo were heartwarming. I loved watching my husband laugh until tears rolled down his face — well, to see that, I'd stick two Kleenex up my nose any day.

I drove home feeling pretty well. I took the biggest stone off the coffee table and threw it into the ocean. Now there were only two small stones left on the table. Oh boy! Yea, me! I think I'm ready to bring it on home.

I should have known post-chemo nausea and pain would catch up with me, and during dinner they did. The first evidence of chemical sickness was a flu-like symptom. The heavy dosages were worse, but the reactions to milder dosages were similar to flu — achy joints, headaches and vague nausea.

I picked up Norman Cousins's book *Anatomy of an Illness* and went to bed. I read how healing laughter can be. He had rented comedy movies to play in his hospital room so he could laugh his way back to health. He laughed long into the night, causing other patients to complain. Laughter *is* healing. Sometimes it's hard to laugh, but with Alan, I never had difficulty. The same was true of Michelle. When I was with Michelle, even though I was getting the dreaded chemotherapy, we laughed a great deal, Charlie, Michelle, and I.

Thursday Alan was leaving for New England, but he would drive me to Bernard's for a table treatment. It would be his last visit for six weeks. I told Alan I hoped Jimmy would spend some time with me. I knew he would be lonely without Alan.

Alan planned to spend his weekends in New York and had arranged to see an old and dear friend of ours there. Bobby was an actor, singer and dancer, wonderful at all three. He had terrible health problems, so I took a crystal pendant from my jewel box to send to him via Alan. I wanted Bobby to have the protection of a crystal over his heart. I also intended to send him a copy of Jaffe's book *Healing from Within*. Bobby was kind to my boys when they were young. In those days he was young, fit. Bobby loved children. He baked huge chocolate cakes, which Jason, Valentine, and Paul devoured with gusto. He was Tante Bobby to my sons. Jason, who heard us call him Tante, thought we were saying Tonto. He was always "Tonto" to Jason. And now I wanted to send a little bit of love to him in New York, where I knew he was having a terrible time.

27

THE DAY AFTER MY SIXTH chemotherapy I was miserable, red-hot the whole day, my face scarlet. It was strange how a terrible heat came over me. Michelle said other patients told her they'd experienced the same thing, so I knew it was the chemotherapy. I hoped it wouldn't get worse. I wondered how much hotter I could get after two more treatments. Each treatment made me boil and I stayed hot throughout the entire three weeks between each therapy.

My agent called and asked me to come to his office. A producer had expressed interest in me, he said. I put him off until the next week. I told him this week was "cooked." It was a funny word to use, and I don't think he knew what I was talking about. I wanted him to think cooked meant busy. Actually, that's how I felt — cooked — red-hot.

The whole week was miserable. I had fevers and chills at five-minute intervals all day and night. For five days it was difficult to sleep. My face, neck and shoulders turned bright red. My hair was soaked and my body bathed in perspiration. It was a miserable, restricting condition.

I had dreadful pain in my right ovary. I called Michael. He said chemotherapy often had a cumulative effect and this seemed to be what was happening to me. He didn't think I should worry about the pain in my ovary, because chemotherapy could irritate ovaries.

I called Ray Weston. After listening sympathetically, he said, "Why don't you take two Ascriptin, dear."

Nobody had answers. I just had to sweat it out — literally. I drank as much water as I could hold. I wanted to drink ten glasses a day, but because I was nauseated, I managed only six. I hoped to flush all the chemicals out of my body. I also stopped meditating. I just couldn't concentrate. However, by the following Sunday, I was better. I woke up knowing I had turned the corner until chemo seven. I got up and for the first time in a long while — at least since I'd suffered the phlebitis — I did some stretching exercises and a few leg lifts. It was a start. Okay, I was going to climb out of this one more time. Here we go again. Up, up and away.

I meditated Sunday and looked forward to the coming week. For the first time in five days I was cheerful and optimistic. My beach house bedroom looked across the veranda out to the ocean through a large picture window. This was a beautiful, late October, bright, sunny day. The ocean was calm and sparkling. Its being Sunday, there were all manner of activities. A kayak race was in progress, and I watched the participants paddling away before my eyes as I sat luxuriating in bed, sipping tea. A funny little airplane flew past the veranda with the pilot looking as if he were pedaling, but of course he wasn't. It was a strange, open-seated craft with canvas wings in bright red and green, almost like something in an animated cartoon. The pilot was perched precariously, open to the elements. If he had turned around and looked at me, I would have offered him some tea — he flew that close to the veranda. The day promised to be entertaining and colorful.

I would attend a horse show in the afternoon where Zuleika was showing again. We had gone the previous day, Saturday. I was sick but I had taken pleasure in watching my daughter win three firsts and three thirds.

We were in a hurry after leaving the beach late. Charlie sped down the road until I said, "Quick, get in the slow lane, I'm going to throw up." He swerved to the side of the road and stopped. I flung open the door, threw up, mopped my brow, slammed the door and said, "Let's go." We made it in time for Zuleika's classes, and the rest of the day was fun.

The barn for which Zuleika rode was full of nice people. Her trainer's daughter, Rainie Rose, was six and had entered her very first walk-trot class and won a ribbon. Rainie was proud and now she organized a show for people around the tack room door. She placed all sorts of objects on the ground — horse liniment, cans of hoof dressing, helmets, sticks — as obstacles to be jumped by the many victims she had lined up. Some were horse-show fathers, Charlie among them. I had the pleasure of watching my husband, on foot, jump the obstacles, competing in Rainie's horse show.

After she'd put them through their paces, Rainie declared it a flat class and Charlie was now entered on foot in a walk, trot and canter. His gaits were judged by Rainie. I loved it. I watched Charlie simulating a horse trotting and then cantering, on the correct lead, of course. Then Rainie announced sitting trot. Charlie bent both knees and trotted in a squatting position. Everyone roared with laughter at this wonderful sight, and Charlie was declared the winner of the class for his sitting trot alone.

"Come here, Rainie," I said, "and sit on my lap and give me a hug." It felt good. Little round, plump, blond, pink and white Rainie, a real horse-show gypsy. She was growing up on horse-show grounds. Everybody knew and loved her.

I was tireless all day, full of energy and having a good time. Dressed in my jeans, Day-Glo yellow socks and matching sweatshirt, with a huge brown felt cowboy hat on my head, I schooled Zuleika and chased around after her on her horse, as I had in the old days. I was happy to be feeling like myself. Everyone covered his or her eyes in pretended blindness at the brightness of my socks and shirt. I loved it. I was back on my feet and looking forward to two more weeks of feeling well.

Next morning I stretched, singing as I jumped into a Day-Glo pink sweatshirt, blue jeans and matching Day-Glo pink socks rolled over my sneakers. I called Cassie and went out on the street to my twenty-year-old Corvette. As I removed the protective cover, I got a wolf whistle and a "Hey, that's a hot pink," from a kid on a bike as he rode by. Hmmm. Not too bad for an old woman. I piled Cassie in the back and warmed up my old friend. I usually took the Jeep for excursions into town because there was more room for Cassie and I did so like her company. When I thought the Corvette was warm enough, I turned on the radio and put my foot down heavily as was my habit in the Jeep. Consequently, I left the curb a streak of Day-Glo pink at sixty miles per hour.

The old car felt good today. She was hot to trot. She had a good radio, and I whizzed down Pacific Coast Highway, singing at the top of my lungs with Anne Murray, and oldie but goodie. Hey, hey, hey baby, I wanna know-o-o-o if I can be your girl, Pa-ba-boom, pa-pa-boom, pa-pa-boom. Shades of the sixties. I was so exhilarated I made a fist à la Dr. Carl Simonton to anchor the great feeling and opened the Vette to eighty in celebration. Whee-ee. Looking good.

Suddenly, out of my elderly car radio came the Eagles singing "Take it to the limit one more time." It really moved me, called to an inner voice I'd been prudently ignoring. But today I was in no mood to be prudent. Take it to the limit one more time.

I put my foot down on the accelerator and drove determinedly to Cross Creek to the stables. I pulled into the entrance. The place seemed deserted. All was quiet. No one was riding in either of the two exercise rings. Great!

My hear beat with excitement and fear as I made straight for Cadok's stall.

"C'mon, Doc-Doc."

I spoke to him reassuringly, calming myself as well as the big, spooky chestnut. As I led him from the stall and into the grooming area, I fastened him in the cross ties, then unlocked the tack room door. I looked furtively around to see if anyone was about, mainly Sue, my secretary, or some other responsible adult who might try to discourage me from what I planned to do. All the time the Eagles were singing in my head. Okay. All right. I'm going for it. I'll take it to my limit one more time, then maybe pack it in. I hoped no one would turn up. I needed my moment of truth and I wanted to have it alone.

I took out my old Hermes saddle and ran my thumb over the small sterling silver nameplate affixed at the back of the seat: *Jill Bronson,* although it was mostly Zuleika's small rump that had sat in it for the past two years. I placed the saddle on top of my tack trunk, then found Cadok's bridle, the old show bridle with the rubber snaffle bit I'd used the last time I'd shown him. He was watching me knowingly from the cross ties.

Taking a soft brush I groomed him in preparation for putting on his saddle. Rubbing some mucus out of his eyes with my thumbs, I told him softly he was a handsome devil. Then I put on his saddle, leaving the bridle until the last minute.

Hunting in the bottom of my trunk, I pulled out my navy blue leather chaps with the name *Jill* done in needlepoint at the back of the waist. I did them up with some difficulty. Bending down and pulling up the zipper was painful on the right side. But I managed. Next I buckled on my spurs. Now I was ready.

So, with one last big breath to dispel all tension I slipped Cadok's bridle over his head and adjusted the buckles. Then I climbed on my tack box and from its top I hopped onto his back. It seemed to me that Cadok tippy-toed out of the enclosed barn area and into the sunlit ring. I must have passed on my feelings of caution and secrecy. But we were out now.

I looked at the ring and fences. They were all set at a height of maybe three and a half feet. But to me they looked like mountains. The small pole we had trotted over previously was no more than a foot high, hardly a jump at all. I wondered what it would feel like to gallop over a fence with one breast gone. Would my instinct to protect myself impede my riding? Would it hurt? Would I fall off? I had to find out.

I warmed Cadok up and then picked up a canter. He pricked his ears. I could feel him listening to me. He was with me. I kept hearing the Eagles in my head. I knew if I didn't take it to the limit now I never would. So I gave Cadok an encouraging squeeze with both my legs and a small jab from my spurs to ensure his continued concentration and cooperation, then I started toward a low white gate.

We jumped it.

Oh, the relief! We made it!

I felt nothing. No pain. No anything. It was as if I'd never been ill. Cadok obviously enjoyed it, so he felt fine, too. I decided this was it, now or never.

I picked up the pace, singing to myself as we galloped around the ring, jumping every fence available to us — the brush box, the triple combination, the gate again, the coop. It was as if neither of us had ever been injured. I was exhilarated and at one with my horse. We jumped everything in the ring once. Then I pulled him up. As I did, I realized I was trembling all over, maybe from relief or fatigue. Then I wondered how I was going to get off the horse.

I sat on Cadok feeling alone and sad, knowing that we would never do this again. I stroked his soft neck and walked him slowly around the ring in the sunshine, thinking things over, glad I'd enjoyed the sensation of jumping that wonderful old horse one more time, glad I had proved to myself I could still do it. I wasn't chicken. Now I could give it up.

Maybe Chakrapani had been right. I patted Cadok's neck.

"Thank you, Doc-Doc. Thank you for all the good times."

I walked him back into the barn and, taking my left foot out of the stirrup, I swung my right leg over the saddle and jumped down to the ground as I'd done a million times. On this occasion, however, I badly scraped my right side on the saddle as I dismounted.

"Ouch!"

Oh, God, it shocked me. As the pain waves shot through my body I leaned my head on Cadok and waited for them to pass, vulnerable again. Then I removed Cadok's saddle, gingerly. I was just about to remove his bridle when my groom

Chewy arrived. He was surprised to see me standing there with the horse. I was glad to see him.

"Chewy, he was such a good boy. But I'm a bit tired. Will you please put him away for me?"

Chewy led Cadok off while I slowly unzipped my chaps, then folded them painstakingly into a small, compact square and locked them in my tack box once again.

I drove home with my mind in a nice quiet place. No thoughts. No questions. No fears. Just a nice, quiet mind. It was a great feeling.

We spent most of the week looking at houses, finding a couple we liked. We had been looking since I told the Skinners to shove it, so to speak, but we hadn't liked anything until now, when suddenly there were three choices. Now it was feast instead of famine. We had choices. The power had shifted. The House That Jack Built was no longer *the* house I wanted, but only one of several possibilities. Oh, hey, hey baby, I wanna kno-o-o if I can be your girl. I made another fist. Fiddle-de-dee, in three weeks I am going back to Tara.

28

IT WAS NOW NOVEMBER 2, five months to the day since my surgery. The next day was Charlie's birthday. I had bought him a red, white and blue trail bike so he could go riding with Paul, Valentine and his son, Tony. The boys had helped me pick out the bike. Paul was to deliver it at one in the morning so I could surprise Charlie the next day. Paul was nervous about it and made me promise if Charlie heard him in the front garden in the middle of the night, I would stop Charlie from shooting him.

I tried to stay awake until the appointed hour so I could see the bike arrive, but I fell asleep. I woke at 5:30 and went downstairs to have a look and to leave a couple of other gifts by Charlie's chair. The bike sat waiting, gleaming on the front patio. Paul had taken the trouble to festoon the bike gaily with balloons and ribbons. Good old Paul; he thought of everything. Among the gifts I left on Charlie's chair was a large amethyst quartz. Purple is a healing color, and this quartz was a lovely deep purple and powerful-looking. I hoped it would keep him healthy and mentally harmonized. I made myself a cup of tea and watched dawn break on Charlie's birthday.

I reflected on how much better I was. How in the beginning when I learned I had cancer, I felt so isolated and alone most of the time. Even when people talked to me, trying to help, their words were like little pebbles pattering on the outside of my body. I was so locked in with my fear nothing penetrated. Now I was better. The terror monster hadn't visited me for ages. I was feeling much more in control.

I still hadn't taken the bone and liver scans, and if I could help it, I wouldn't. My periods had stopped. I always had been regular before, twenty-eight days by the calendar, but after chemo number three, they stopped completely. Michael told me this often happened with drugs. My gynecologist wanted to check out the nagging pain in my right ovary, but I told him I would wait until chemotherapy was over. If the pain wasn't caused by the drugs, they probably couldn't do anything about it while I was having treatments. If it were, I assumed the symptoms would disappear when I stopped being pumped full of drugs. Then maybe my periods would come back or maybe they wouldn't. Michael said they might not, as I was approaching menopause. I had always dreaded my periods stopping; it made me sad to think of it. Although I didn't intend having more children, the thought that one day I would no longer have a choice saddened me. It was like the beginning of the end. But now that I hadn't menstruated for three months, I found I didn't miss it at all. Quite the contrary, I hoped my periods wouldn't start again. I didn't feel less a woman after all. I realized there was no doubt about it — nope, none at all. I was a woman. With or without menstruation or with one or two breasts. I was born a woman and that was the way I was going to stay.

I had about a quarter of an inch of hair regrowth in all the bald patches. It was short, but no longer as thin, and no scalp was showing anymore. As I sipped my tea, I felt at peace. I had made mental progress and now my hair was growing back. True, I needed more exercise. I made an early morning resolution that I would ride Cadok tomorrow. I also determined to walk every day.

My confidence was up most of the time. Meditation was still difficult. Sometimes it would be good; sometimes my mind would drift about and concentration on the visualizations was almost impossible. In spite of that, it worked. I had changed my beliefs about my disease. Every day for the past five months I had told myself that cancer was a weak disease composed of weak, confused cells. I had constructed a new belief system: I was stronger than my cancer cells. I had to admit to a certain amount of pride. I had come through the last five months. I had to face two more chemos. If nothing unforeseen happened, I would be home and dry by Christmas. The family would be together in Vermont. I could start the New Year fresh with this all behind me. Another new start.

We went to a Mexican restaurant to celebrate Charlie's birthday — Suzanne, Tony, Paul, Valentine, Katrina and Zuleika, with Charlie at the head of the table and me on his right. The party was fun with all the family. Missing was Jason, whose car broke down on his way to the beach. He turned up later at the house with a gift for Charlie, a girlfriend and an empty stomach. Katrina and I made a huge omelet for him and his girlfriend, Rena. Zuleika, Katrina, Jason and Rena sat around the kitchen table chatting, while Charlie and Tony visited in the sitting room. The others had gone home. Before he left, Tony, a deepy religious Catholic, told me, "I disagree with some of the means you're seeking for cures. I'm sure if you pray to Our Lady, she will help you." Then, saying, "You are in all my prayers," he gave me a hug and kissed me good night. Charlie had received a nice collection of gifts, some pertaining to his new trail bike, and some toys: a large fist on a string, which Paul gave him along with a motorcycle helmet; a toy airplane to use on the beach from Jason; two sweaters from Suzanne; goggles from Zuleika, and a throwing knife from Katrina. Valentine bought a waist pouch for Charlie to wear while he was biking and — whoops — Tony gave him a motorcycle helmet. Charlie enjoyed his day. He piled his loot around his desk, where it remained for many more days before we left the house for Bel Air.

I had one more week before my next treatment, and, as was my pattern, I became anxious. Everyone said "only two more," but to me it was *two* more — each one an experience of its own. There was no *only* about it. Sue Colin tried to get me to relax. I told her I could not afford to relax my vigilant eye. I had to be careful or the next chemo might be the one that got me.

"So you still feel it might finish you off?" she asked.

"Yup." The terrible heat after chemo six had been a big test of my strength. I told Sue I had to fight the heat the way I had fought the Compazine reaction. I couldn't give in to it; I had to fight.

She asked if I could think of it as a healing energy. "Remember," she said, "heat is energy."

"No. It is too hot. If I meditated or put my mind down into the heat, it would fry and zap it up, rather like freeze-dried coffee."

Sue laughed and said I had one helluva imagination, but I persisted and said the only way I could handle it was to be stoic and withstand, to use my strength to fight it so I didn't burn up. Another method I used was to remove my mind from my body and let the whole thing go on without me.

She said, "But I don't want you to leave your body."

"Oh, I'm not leaving for good. I'll be coming back. Is that spooky?"

Sue said she would like to see if I could find a way to accept the feeling.

"No, I can't. It's too hot." I told her people with catastrophic diseases dealt with them in different ways. Some didn't want to talk about their disease, some couldn't stop talking about it, some gained insight and tremendous wisdom, and some used it as a giveaway to help others. Some became bitter and angry, and some gave up. Some fought.

Sue asked me to close my eyes and relax. She led me through a meditation, asking me to think of the energy of the earth coming up through my feet and through my whole body, then to take my mind to a place where I felt secure, happy and energized. My mind went straight to the barn. She told me to touch a place on my hand to anchor this feeling. I immediately put two fingers of my right hand into my left as

Dr. Simonton had taught me. This was the symbol he used to anchor peace and love feelings, just as the right-hand fist was an anchor for power feelings. She had me scan my body for tension. I used one of my white blood cells as a scanner. I sent it down to my toes, up my legs and all over my body. It was a good meditation and I did feel relaxed and energized afterward. She gave me a big hug when I left. Sue is a therapist who touches her patients — another important thing, I think, to touch people with isolating illness or disease. Once you get used to it, a hug or a touch can be so comforting. Being ill, fighting a disease is isolating and lonely and, quite simply — as the bumper stickers say — a hug helps.

I drove home in good spirits in time to have lunch and leave again with Charlie for Michael's office for my midtreatment blood test prior to chemo seven. Today, there were dishes of candy left over from Halloween lying around the office. I resisted. I had my blood test and told Michael, "I don't suppose there's any way I could talk you into cutting down my chemo?"

"Why?"

"Well, because last time I got so hot that I fear, with the cumulative effect, I'll get so hot I won't be able to stand it."

"Sorry, Jill. Unless your white blood cells are down too far, I'm afraid I'm going to be hard."

"Give me a moment or two to meditate," I joked. "I'll see what I can do." I also discussed the painful ovary with him and a pain around my liver. Michael examined my liver, pressing hard into my side. No pain on examination, so it was probably an offshoot from the pain in my ovary.

"Michael, can I ask you something? If I have cancer anywhere in my body, will this chemo get rid of it?"

"Now, understand, Jill, we're not worried about any other cancer, only the possibility of the original breast cancer metastasizing somewhere else. And it could be anywhere, even places we haven't thought of. If it has, hopefully [Michael always said "hopefully"] this treatment will get it."

I was very strong that day to be able to hold that conversation. However, as I left the office, I did two things. I made the appointment for my seventh chemotherapy in six days' time and I took a handful of Halloween candy and ate it in the elevator going down to the street.

"Charlie," I said as I slid into the car, "I didn't know there was a possibility of a tumor existing somewhere else in my body."

"Yes, you did. That's why you wouldn't take the bone and liver scans."

"Oh, yes, I suppose I did. But today is the first time I've really talked about it." I always talked about a stray cell maybe attaching and growing someplace in the future, but I'd never discussed the possibility that I was even now harboring another tumor. Well, until today I hadn't been ready to deal with that.

That night Alan called from his film's location on Cape Cod. He had made friends with one of the actors in the movie. He learned the actor had a young wife with cancer who was going through chemotherapy. Alan told him about our friendship and my experiences. The actor asked Alan if he thought I would call his wife, as he was worried about her being alone. I told Alan of course I would. I knew it could be lonely when your husband was away making a movie, not to mention dealing with illness at the same time. I imagined we had things to say to each other. Alan and I chatted for a while. I told him I missed him. He said, "Oh, I love being missed." He nagged me about my diet before we said good night.

The next day I called the actor's wife. Her name was Willie. She sounded down. Her voice was deep and carried a country twang. We compared notes on therapy, doctors and feelings. Willie's cancer was in her lower intestine. Her surgeon had been unable to remove it all. Willie had a five-month-old daughter. Now she thought she might be pregnant again as she had discovered a small lump in her lower abdomen. She was going to the doctor the next day. She worried that the tumor might be growing. We talked about how all symptoms were cancer to us. She laughed when I told her I'd even had cancer in my pinky. As we laughed, conversation became easier — two strangers with only our disease in common. I had no way of knowing what she looked like; I only related to her voice. We discussed her possible pregnancy. I asked if she had symptoms like swollen breasts, sickness or fatigue. I asked if her nipples had turned brown, always a sure sign of pregnancy with me. She laughed and said she was brown all over.

"Oh, you're black."

"Yes."

We made plans to meet the following Friday. I told her I'd be interested in the results of her visit to the doctor and asked her to call anytime she felt like talking.

I added something new to my daily routine — the *I Ching,* or *Book of Changes,* the main source of inspiration to Confucius and Lao-tzu. It deals with one of the first efforts of the human mind to place itself within the universe and had been used in China for three thousand years. It is a book of oracles, small philosophical parables, which I found interesting and inspiring, evoked with the help of three coins and my trusty *I Ching Work Book.*

There are many ways to read the *I Ching.* One involves counting fifty yarrow stalks from the plant *Achillea millefolium.* Another involves six wands, colored beads, preprogrammed calculators and computers! I found it simpler, however, to use the more common method of tossing three coins in the air. I cupped the pennies in my hand, shook them, and let them drop on a flat surface. The first fall represents the bottom line of a hexagram. I do this six times, each fall representing another line in the hexagram, which I then take to my *Book of Changes* to find my Chinese advice of the day.

I would throw the coins in the morning. Today I was getting a wonderful "present situation" and an oppressive "future direction of the present." Oh, heck. However, it did make sense. I was feeling good right now, but my future week would be oppressive because of my seventh chemo on Monday.

As the week progressed, I developed a nervous stomach anticipating the next treatment. I had reached a saturation point with the cumulative effect of chemicals. I smelled trouble. As if to confirm my intuition, a large ulcer developed on the side of my bottom lip. I wished Michael would cut down the dose, while, at the same time, I wanted to receive the full measure to ensure that we'd killed all the cancer.

Bernard told me I was doing really well as far as he could see. He thought all the cancer was gone. He had developed a new liquid with vitamins and minerals in an alcohol base. I took it four times a day, along with the water that had had an electric current run through it. All Bernard's patients were now carrying two brown dropper bottles, one with charged water and the other with the new mixture. Sue Colin told me she felt energized by the vitamins and I had to confess so did I. Bernard told me the mixture was curing all kinds of illnesses. He thought he had cracked it, as he put it. I found him a fascinating person. Sue thought he was a genius. I didn't know about that, but something kept me going.

I was looking good, feeling good, and my hair, though still short, had almost completely grown back. I had a wonderfully robust appetite. In fact, people told me I looked the picture of health. I was doing all the right things. I had therapy to help change my cancer personality and to help deal with fear. I took the table regularly and I meditated. I was also having chemotherapy and regular medical checkups. Now if I could just get through the next two years without a recurrence. Henceforth, time was going to be my friend. No longer was I going to hate each year that went by, feeling it was making me older and older. In the future, as time went by with no recurrence, I was going to feel younger.

The day before my chemo, Katrina was with friends and Sue Overholt had taken Zuleika to a horse show. I stayed home, contentedly sharing the house and ocean with Charlie.

It was hot on the veranda. The large, round orange float on which I relaxed was comfortable. I was drowsy. Charlie read, sitting in the shade of the umbrella, which was open over the round table on which we had lunch. I looked over at my husband. His body was tanned and strong, his eyes squinted in the glare as he read the paper without glasses. His legs, with the strong calf muscles, were crossed, one foot tapping out a silent rhythm. I looked at his foot. I had once told Charlie he had gentleman's feet. They are beautiful, smooth with golden skin, well proportioned, no calluses or bunions. He has large, well-formed toenails. Looking at his nails, my mind went daydreaming off to another time.

Many years earlier we were staying at the Grand Hotel Brighton in England. My father was recuperating from major intestinal surgery and we were there to visit him. Zuleika was only five and she had been given her first bottle of clear nail polish so she could be like Mommy. Zuleika was into painting nails. She had done her own and mine. Now she was looking for another victim. She had been eyeing her father's nails for some time. He was reading the paper, as he was now, barefoot, one leg crossed. Finally she asked, "Daddy, can I paint your toenails, please?"

Charlie put down the paper and smiled at her. He always found it hard to deny Zuleika anything. She stood there with the bottle of transparent polish. It looked innocent enough. "Sure you can, baby." Charlie went back to his paper. Carefully, Zuleika painted Charlie's big toenail with the clear varnish. He inspected it. "Hmm, looks like chicken fat's been smeared on it."

"Daddy!" Zuleika was insulted.

"No, I'm joking, baby, carry on." Charlie disappeared once more behind the paper.

Watching this tableau, I couldn't resist! Putting one finger over my lips to caution Zuleika not to react, I started painting his other foot with bright red polish. It really showed up well on Charlie's big square nails. I gave the bottle to Zuleika. She delightedly went over the clear top coat with the sparkling paint. Soon, Charlie had a matched set of ten bright red toenails. Engrossed in his paper, he seemed to forget what we were doing. We tidied up and put the bottles away. I tried hard not to giggle. Zuleika, on the other hand, seeing no reason why her father should not have red toenails, was proud of the finished result. She couldn't wait for him to discover our handiwork. "Daddy, look at your toes."

He looked down. "You didn't tell me you were going to paint them red. Where did you get that varnish?"

"It's a surprise, Daddy. Mummy gave it to me. Doesn't it look good?"

Charlie wiggled his toes, looking long and hard at them. "How do you get it off?"

I gave him a big smile. "You wait for it to wear off. I think they look very nice."

Charlie narrowed his eyes. "How long does that take? Don't you have that stuff to take it off?"

"No, I don't," I lied.

Zuleika was excited. "Daddy, they look so good. Can I put flowers on them? Mummy's got lots of colors. I'll paint pale pink flowers on top of the red. You've got such nice big nails. I can do it easily. Please, Daddy?"

Charlie, seeing her pleasure, melted. He gave her a big grin. "Sure you can, baby, go ahead."

The next hour was devoted to the decorating of Charlie's toenails. A pale silver pink was used to make small roses on his right big toe, and a deeper pink made for a daisy on his left. It was quite a sight. Charlie sat patiently, keeping his feet carefully still while the roses dried. Zuleika surveyed her artwork and declared the pedicure complete.

It was close to teatime. Today, we were going to have tea with Grandma and Grandpa, as Zuleika called my parents, at their home in Seaford, Sussex. It was to be Zuleika's second visit to their home. The first time, a few days previously, had been very special. My parents had been sitting framed by the big front window of their living room, waiting for us to arrive. To her, the small cottage and pretty garden with the path leading to the door were like a scene from *The Blue Bird,* the one in which Shirley Temple visits her grandparents in her dreams — it is every little girl's idea of where a "grandma" and "grandpa" should live. To complete the fantasy, two white-haired, picture-book grandparents were sitting, looking out the window, happily awaiting her arrival. They certainly made a fuss over Zuleika. On her first visit she was the star, Charlie the co-star and I was merely a supporting player.

We all sat down and had a proper English tea: cucumber, watercress, tomato and ham and cheese finger sandwiches, fruitcake, biscuits (cookies to most Americans) and, of course, Indian tea with milk and sugar. Then my father, who was well along in his recovery and feeling full of vigor, took Zuleika outside into the garden, gave her a plastic ball and small bat and the two of them started a game. My mother saw her opportunity and brought out the scrapbooks.

I covered my face with my hands. "Oh, God, no, Mummy." But it was too late. They had been put ceremoniously on a small table in front of my husband. The books held press clippings and photographs. Charlie looked carefully through my baby photographs, noticing a resemblance between me and Zuleika at the same age. He browsed through my early press clippings, politely turning the pages. Then suddenly he stopped. He looked quizzically at me, then back at the page, then at me again. The picture that demanded his attention was my Easter still, circa 1962. Back then, every Easter and Christmas I was photographed in appropriate costume. All the contract players at Rank had pictures taken during those holidays for publicity purposes. The photograph that caught Charlie's eye was of me dressed in a chicken outfit — a yellow feathered, strapless leotard and a feathered skullcap. I was in my ballet shoes, posed on one leg, balanced on the point of one shiny yellow slipper, one leg coyly bent. I looked very young and very embarrassed. I was standing incongruously beside a giant broken egg. It was meant to suggest I had just been hatched. My head was on one side and I was wearing what I had hoped was a sexy expression. This was a pout and an imbecilic, sly sidelong glance. My eyes were doing their best to smolder. I looked crazed; the whole effect was absurd. Charlie started to laugh.

"What?" My mother stiffened. To her, the books were serious stuff. "What are you laughing at, Charles? I wouldn't have shown you if I'd known you were going to laugh."

By now, tears were rolling down Charlie's cheeks. He couldn't stop. "Oh, Jesus, Jill, this is so funny. A chicken oufit. I can't believe it. Jesus, it's so funny!"

My mother put her glasses on and took a closer look. "What are you laughing at? She looks lovely."

I was laughing, too. "Oh, Mummy, I could have told you he'd laugh. Now I'll never live it down. He'll never let me forget it."

My father came in with Zuleika. "What's going on?"

This brought fresh laughter from my husband. The tone of the afternoon was deteriorating rapidly. So I took my reluctant daughter and still-laughing husband back to the hotel. We would meet my mother and father tomorrow in Brighton, far away from all the old scrapbooks.

The next day while mother, Zuleika and I wandered down the century-old Brighton lanes, Charlie and my father scuttled off to buy some shirts. They get along well. Daddy was happy and proud to be with his famous son-in-law. During their walk Charlie saw some sandals he liked. They entered the elegant British shoe store. A man in a dark suit approached them. Charlie pointed to the shoes he wanted. The assistant, very proper, very English and courteous, brought him the brown leather sandals. Charlie sat down and kicked off his shoes, too late remembering his naked, sockless feet. You could have heard a pin drop as the shoe salesman and my father looked down at the red toenails with the roses and daisies winking up at them.

Inscrutably, Charlie looked up at them looking down at his toes. There was a long silence. The shop assistant inspected the nails for a moment longer. Then, with an arch smile, he said, "Sweet!" My father was speechless. He couldn't believe his eyes, and for the first time in his life, words failed him.

Charlie asked quietly, "Do I need socks to try on the shoes?" which broke the spell. Charlie doesn't like to explain. The sandals were tried on and paid for without further comment. Carrying his new package, Charlie walked nonchalantly out of the store, followed by my incredulous father.

The two men joined us in the small park where we had agreed to meet. My father couldn't wait to tell us what had happened. Sitting on the bench, he related in an amazed voice, "Then you could have knocked me down with a feather. Charles took off his shoes, and his toenails were painted RED." He shook his head in disbelief as he told my mother. Zuleika butted in with glowing pride.

"I did them, Grandpa, aren't they great? Would you like me to do yours?"

Her grandfather politely, but definitely, declined. The polish stayed on Charlie's nails for weeks. He patiently waited for it to wear off. I liked the fact that it didn't bother him, and Zuleika loved it. It became, over the weeks, quite commonplace to us. When we left England and went to conservative Spain, the room service waiter at the hotel was rendered incapable of movement and speech for at least sixty seconds the day Charlie prowled into the sitting room of the suite where dinner was being set up. Fresh from his shower, Charlie was barefoot, wearing a robe. Oblivious to the man's astonishment, he signed the check, tipped the waiter, then, saying "Buenos noches," he sat calmly down to eat. It was too much for the Latin mentality. The old waiter couldn't believe his eyes. There was Charles Bronson, macho hombre, sitting there with his wife and child, calmly eating his dinner with scarlet toenails. He backed out of the room, still staring, bumping the door with his shoulder as he left, not even thanking Charlie for the tip or saying "Buenos noches" in return. My husband with his gentleman's feet.

I lay there on the veranda overlooking the sea a while longer, enjoying, remembering. Those had been happy years when Zuleika was a small child. Then I got up from my float and gave Charlie a kiss. "Let's take a little walk, darling. Would you like to?" Umhumm. He returned my kiss. We left the veranda and walked down the beach. I held his arm as we strolled, watching Cassie try to catch the sandpipers. She loved it when we both took her for a walk. I had a mellow feeling. I would always have my memories. As we walked, I realized this moment of tranquility and peace would be added to my memory bank to be called on and reenjoyed whenever I needed it. I made a fist to anchor it.

We returned to the house and sat for a while, watching the huge crashing waves that the full moon always brought. The tide was coming in, the beach was disappearing and the ocean was washing under the house supports. I loved it when the waves rushed under the house. It was almost like being on a boat. We only had one more week here in the rented house. I knew I would miss it.

29

THE NEXT DAY I RECEIVED a large, fat envelope from Cape Cod. It contained a furry, little beige toy dog that had been somewhat squashed in the mail, and a letter from Alan. The letter read:

Here I am in the makeup trailer, bored to death. I wish I was with you, driving along in Granny, heading for Bernard's, but I need the money, so here I am. How I wish I was a little richer and maybe not quite so much of a beauty. This has always been a curse — my beauty, that is. I wish I could tell you how I know deep down inside that you are going to be feeling really good, better than you have felt in a long time. It's the last mile now, honey. Then it's home free and clear — a whole new, wonderful, healthy life. That's what's in store for you. Just try to hang on to those thoughts when you are feeling low; and for goodness sake, don't expect so much of yourself. Be kind to Jill. I think about you a great deal, and whenever I do, it's with a wonderful, warm feeling. I wish I could tell you what a wonderful being you are and how rich and full I feel from knowing you; but, instead, all I seem to do is put down dreary bullshit. Somehow you will have to piece it together. But, sweetie, know in your gut things are going to be great. *I* know it. And don't let that feeling go away. Before you realize it, this will all be over and we will be laughing and carrying on as usual. Say hello to Charlie and family and a big kiss for Cassie. Love to you, Alan.

P.S. I sent you that watchdog to see that you stay on your diet.

Everyone should have an Alan in her life.

Alan had asked his friend King Zimmerman to substitute for him, and the next morning King came by to take me to Bernard's and then to lunch. Cassie didn't quite accept King. (He had often been in the car with Alan and me and had always sat in the backseat with Cassie. I think Cassie believed King was Alan's dog!) She definitely lorded it over poor King. While I was upstairs at Bernard's lying on the table, King volunteered to take Cassie for a walk. But she showed no interest, wouldn't go with him and jumped into the backseat, refusing even to look at him.

After lunch, King drove me home and I took a short nap before Charlie and I left for Beverly Hills and chemo seven. I was very, very tired and had great discomfort around the right side of my diaphragm, the incision and in my armpit. I wondered if I could attribute the fatigue to the hours on Bernard's table. In any event, about two-thirty, Charlie and I took off for Michael's office.

I told Michael, "I'm very tired." I took my blood test and showed him the sore on my lip and said the hot sweats had diminished somewhat in the past week. We went into one of the rooms where I usually received my chemotherapy. He gave me a paper gown and left the room. I took off my shirt, my bra and my right breast.

"This is some fancy robe you gave me, Michael," I said on his return. "It has no armholes." I'd wrapped it around myself.

He gently probed the scar. I found myself fascinated by the long, straight gray hairs standing up in his curly brown mop. I gave in to an impulse and pulled one out, much to his irritation.

"When you've finished!" He paused in his probing, then listened with his stethoscope. "Is there any pain when you breathe in?" He had me take a few deep breaths.

"Yes, there is some."

His fingers found a swelling to the right of my scar. "There is some fluid here, Jill. I don't think there's any reason for concern. But if it doesn't go away soon, I would want you to have an X ray. For the time being, though, we won't worry about it. I also feel you shouldn't have your chemotherapy today. I've learned to respect your feelings about what your body tells you. You've been right almost all the time. If you tell me, as you did last week, that you feel you've reached capacity, I think you need more time. It's not uncommon, when you've had chemotherapy as long as you have, to spread out the last few. Right now, you're full of it."

I told him, "You're right. I feel as if it's up to here," putting my hand across the bridge of my nose.

He raised his hand even higher and said, "I think at this point, it's more like up to here."

Charlie was disappointed. We had calculated that if I had chemotherapy today, the eighth and last treatment would be three weeks before Christmas, thereby giving me a full ten days before we flew to Vermont for the holidays. Also, the following Monday we were leaving for Santa Barbara for a horse show with Zuleika.

We always spent Thanksgiving in Santa Barbara. For the last nine years I had shown at what we called the Turkey Show. The whole family gathered; it was something we enjoyed. My chemotherapy was delayed until the following Monday — one full week — which meant I would have to go immediately thereafter to Santa Barbara. Also, more worry to Charlie. It didn't give me enough time to recover properly before leaving for Vermont. We left Michael's office and drove home in a quiet, depressed mood.

I was worried about Charlie. This whole thing hadn't been much fun for him, and I could see he was beginning to feel the pressure. I believe he was as locked in by my illness as I. I wished he'd go out and have some fun. I tried to talk him into taking a ski trip while Zuleika, Sue Overholt and I went to Santa Barbara, but he said, "No. I'm committed to this until it's over, just as you are." Somehow, I felt more concerned and worried about Charlie's state of mind at that point than I did my own.

At home Cassie jumped joyously around me, and when I turned my back to her to look out at the sea, she jumped to my shoulders with her feet. Then, when she couldn't get the kind of attention she sought, she promptly undid both my shoelaces. "What's the matter, girl? What do you want?" She gave me a funny, high-pitched squealing sound and jumped again. I knew she wanted to go for a walk. Well, that wasn't such a bad idea.

Storm clouds had gathered over the ocean. Winter was approaching. I thought perhaps there would be a storm that night. I enjoyed the atmosphere. Moist and overcast, it reminded me of England. Cassie and I took a forty-five-minute walk. When I came back, I did feel better. I found an old towel and rubbed her dry. Even though it was cold, it didn't stop Cassie from galloping through the waves trying to catch the gulls and sandpipers.

We ate dinner quietly, at least Charlie and I did. The girls were in their usual high spirits. Katrina had a little problem with one of her boyfriends, which Zuleika loved to hear about. In fact, the only thing Zuleika enjoyed more than Katrina's stories was to listen in on the extension phone when Katrina spoke to them. I thought this was very generous of Katrina.

Later that night, Alan called from Cape Cod to ask how my chemotherapy had gone. I told him about going, taking my pills and not getting the treatment after all. Alan gave me one of his rallying pep talks.

"Just take one day at a time," he said. "So you're not having it now. It's better that you take your time. You've only got two more. I know you're depressed about it, but everything's going to be okay. Everything's going to be wonderful."

30

ALAN HAD REMINDED ME that that evening the Theresa Saldana story, *Victims for Victims,* was showing on TV. Theresa had been a special project of Hilary's and mine. We felt we had rediscovered her by fighting to have her cast in *The Evil That Men Do* after she had been brutally attacked and slashed on a Los Angeles street. Alan had done her makeup both in that picture and *Victims for Victims.*

Katrina and I sat in the bedroom and watched the show. We had different reactions. Katrina, who had been through her own tragic story and was a victim herself, was angry at scenes in which Theresa was stabbed and nobody came to help. Katrina had been through a similar experience. While her mother lay dying in her arms of a heart attack, she screamed and called for help. It was summer and the windows were open. I was told afterward that people heard but nobody responded. The same thing happened to Theresa, until a Sparkletts water man, Jeff Burke, came to her rescue. Everybody heard, but people gathered around and actually watched her being stabbed. Theresa reenacted the scene very, very well. It made me cry. Katrina's tears were angry ones.

When the drama ended Charlie came upstairs. He knew the story would depress him, so he had watched a ball game instead.

Charlie and I stood at the window watching the ocean pound in. It began to storm heavily. Oh good, I wanted to experience one violent storm at the beach. It didn't look as if it would develop fully that night, but it was rough enough to excite me. We also wanted it to rain heavily on a house we had bid on, a pretty, Spanish house on one floor, just a mile and a half from the beach, and about the same distance to the stables and barn. I had fallen in love with this new home. The house was on a quiet road in a garden with four big old oak trees surrounded by a high Spanish wall. It seemed perfect. We hoped the rainstorm would be strong enough to test the house, which was situated in a state-declared flood area. It had been completed two years earlier, so it hadn't been through much. Would the creek nearby overflow and flood the house? We wanted it christened before we went into escrow, so we would know what we were dealing with.

As for the House That Jack Built, Charlie and I were glad we didn't have to think about it anymore or the pack of lawyers who lived in it. It was a relief putting that experience behind us once and for all.

I told Charlie I was concerned about the painful swelling around my incision and down the side of my body.

Charlie told me not to worry about the swelling in the incision. He reminded me that Michael said he wasn't concerned.

"But it seems to be getting worse."

"Don't worry, baby. If Michael thought it was something to be concerned about, he would have had it X-rayed."

I was depressed and it showed. I didn't bother to wear makeup; every day I just jumped into my gray flight suit. I tried to contact Dr. Simonton. He was just what I needed to pull me out of this slump. However, he wasn't due in California until January. Nothing lifted me out of my doldrums. I arranged to see Dr. Karlan, who was performing a biopsy at a hospital near Sue Colin's office when I reached him. I told him I'd see him the next day, which gave me time to see Sue first.

Feeling puny, I sat huddled in the corner of Sue's couch, curled up with my sweater pulled protectively around me.

She asked, "Well, what is it all about?"

"I feel pressure from all sides. Pressure about leaving the beach house, having to pack and take everything back to Bel Air, pressure at the thought of buying a new house and moving out of Bel Air, which I know is going to be a monumental task. God, just deciding which pieces of furniture to keep and which I want to leave is a job in itself. Then there's storage: paintings, papers, filing cabinets, clothing . . . ."

"Wait a minute, wait a minute. Don't think ahead. What else are you worried about?"

"I'm worried about delaying chemotherapy. It means I'll be having therapy the day before I go to Santa Barbara to watch Zuleika ride."

"Then don't go to Santa Barbara."

"But I want to. I really want to watch Zuleika ride."

"Well, maybe right now you just can't do everything, Jill. Right now, you have to take care of yourself."

"I'm also concerned about Christmas, Sue. I'm worried that I won't be well enough to go to Vermont."

"Do you want to go to Vermont?"

"At this moment, no, I don't. I'm terrified of getting on an airplane, knowing those doors are shut and I'm locked in with no escape. I'm scared I'll panic and not be able to breathe. I get so terribly tired now. It will take us about nine hours to get to Vermont — a five-and-a-half-hour plane ride to Boston and then a three-hour car ride from the airport. It's so cold and there's so much to do when I get there."

"Well, maybe you shouldn't go to Vermont."

"I have to go, Sue. I have no choice. Charlie's looking forward to it. It means so much to him." Sue saw my panic at the thought of disappointing Charlie. She backed off.

"All right, what else is worrying you?"

"I don't know. I know there are only two more chemos, but I'm so tired."

Sue led me through a meditation. She asked me to visualize a white light over my head shining into my head and through my body, to visualize it scanning my body, relaxing and filling me with well-being. As usual, the relaxation did help and I left Sue's feeling somewhat better — not much, but a little.

I went on to the Beverly Hills Medical Center to meet with Mitchell Karlan. He was in surgery when I arrived. He came bustling out, all business.

"Hello, Jill, how are you? Come with me, dear."

He led me, of all places, into the post-operative room. There was a woman patient with her husband and mother, both swathed in green the way Paul and Charlie had been. She was lying on a table waiting to go in for her biopsy, which Mitchell was to perform. He took me to a corner of the room and pulled some curtains around a bed. I removed my sweater and shirt and showed him the incision area.

"Put your arms up, dear, and let me have a look." He closed his eyes as he always did and began deftly feeling around the scar and under my armpit. "Oh, this is doing beautifully. It's healing just beautifully. You're fine. Don't worry about anything. There's nothing wrong here at all."

"But why am I having the swelling and soreness?"

"Well, sometimes when you're using the muscles a bit more than usual, that will happen; I believe you're beginning to get some feeling back in the nerves."

"Then I'm fine. Okay, then there's nothing to worry about?"

He gave me a kiss and said, "No, you're just fine, dear. You're looking great. I want to see you in a month, though."

I thanked him and as I was leaving I saw him go to the lady who awaited her biopsy. He said, "Don't let them put you to sleep until I get back."

I heard her say, "Oh, no, they're going to put me to sleep?"

I left the room in a hurry. I wished I could have done something to reassure her. Had she been having a mastectomy, maybe I would have volunteered. But knowing she was having a biopsy, I thought perhaps I wasn't the right person to speak up.

I returned to the beach and spent the evening sitting on the couch sorting out my feelings about moving away from the sea. The beach house had been good to me all summer and had seen me through some rough times. I suppose it was to be expected that I would be irritable and grumpy about now. Once more I was in a holding pattern. I was waiting for chemo seven on Monday, waiting to find out if I would be well enough to drive to Santa Barbara for Thanksgiving with the family, and waiting to find out if we would get the new house. Our first bid had been turned down, as expected. I didn't know how it would all turn out.

As I lay ruminating on my couch, the telephone rang. I picked it up listlessly, uninterested in speaking to anyone.

"Hello, Jill?"

At first, I didn't recognize the voice that was once so familiar that the next words would have been unnecessary.

"It's David."

David. It was so unexpected. I almost said, "David who?" Then a rush of recognition hit with a series of mental pictures. David sitting at a desk, head cocked, shoulders slightly hunched, wearing a large terry-cloth robe. David deep in a world of his own, his back to the room, conducting the London Symphony Orchestra while hunched over the record player. David, who had known me so intimately. David, my ex-husband, was saying, "How are you doing? I was so sorry to hear you've been having a rough time."

He sounded so nice, very familiar and cozy. I was flustered, taken off guard. This wasn't going to be easy. It was the first time we'd spoken for almost three years.

"Paul called me and told me you'd been unwell."

David, always the master of understatement. Well, I guess getting a tit whacked off and six months of chemotherapy could come under the category of unwell.

"Yes, but I'm doing really well. I'm into holistic healing and meditation. I have what's known as a good attitude."

He said, "Well, you always had that."

"I'm going to be fine. In fact, I feel great. Where are you?"

"I'm calling from Calgary, Canada. I'm up here doing a play. It's very isolated and lonely. I'm practically a monk. I spend all my time in my room reading when I'm not at the theater. It's like being in Siberia. I feel like Solzhenitsyn or something."

"Gosh, David," I said, unaccountably striving for the youthful, enthusiastic voice he'd known way back when. "I have a really good friend in Calgary, one of my old horse-riding cronies, Dessa Davidson. Why don't you call her if you're lonely? She's a lot of fun. Maybe you could have dinner with her. At least call and say hello for me. She's very enter-taining. She can do all of Stanley Holloway's old comedy re-citals in a cockney accent. She'll make you laugh."

David sounded doubtful. "Comedy recitations and a riding buddy, eh?"

"David, really, call her. She's great. She'll cheer you up. She's quite sophisticated and attractive, honestly."

"Okay, tell me the number. Maybe I will."

"How are Katherine and the children?"

"Oh, they're just great." He went on about some of their achievements and activities.

I wanted to say, "Oh, David, I'm so glad you called; it's good to hear your voice. I feel so down. This chemo they are giving me is hell, and, David, I've lost a breast." I wanted to play "Do you remember when?" to recapture our youth, but that conversation belonged to another time, another place. Instead, I said, "Thank you so much for thinking of me. Don't forget to call Dessa. Take care of yourself, David. Say hello to Katherine."

There was a long pause, and then we both said good-bye.

I sank back into my couch. It was nice of him to call. I was filled with nostalgic thoughts. How sweet he'd been — how sweet we'd both been. My thoughts drifted back to the sixties. Cassie's sudden barking on the veranda brought me back to the present. I'm still pretty damn sweet now, I told myself, making a fist. I went out onto the veranda to see why Cassie was barking. Kate, the Doberwoman from next door, was prancing about on the beach, trying to entice Cassie down for a romp. I unlatched the gate and watched them play. It was obvious that the two dogs had developed a close friendship. They would probably miss each other. I wouldn't be the only one to miss the beach.

This was a gloomy time personally, no doubt about it. However, my daughter was flourishing. All Zuleika's hard work was paying off. She was among the top ten riders in the Los Angeles County Finals. Charlie and I attended one of her classes. I could hardly believe it was Zuleika. She looked so tall and fine on Susie Dotan's horse Arrow. Zuleika and Arrow were a fine team. It was exciting and moving to see how my little girl had improved and how mature she was. She showed well against the other girls, some of them as old as eighteen with more experience and mileage. Yep, I thought to myself, the kid's got class.

Charlie, trapped by my illness, would have liked to go skiing or ride his motorcycle or just take a trip and go off somewhere. I wished he would. I felt guilty knowing he was hanging around waiting for me to get well. It put an extra burden on me.

"I can't leave you until you're well," he said. "I just wouldn't feel right."

Oh, my gosh, I had to get well quickly. Everybody would lose their patience.

Even though Dr. Karlan said everything was well with me, I worried about the pain under my incision around my ribs. It was never ceasing; at times I thought I could feel little nodular lumps around the area of pain. I feared it was a thrombosis or phlebitis. My hypochondriacal personality pushed its way to the fore and had a field day.

My father's stroke had occurred four months after surgery and his doctor said he had thrown an embolism due to the surgery. I suspected it would happen to me. My fear of going to Vermont increased day by day. I now added to my general feeling of anxiety the fear that I would have a stroke while I was in our Vermont country house, where the nearest hospital was at least an hour's drive away. I wanted to conquer these fears, but there seemed to be nothing I could do but dance with them, as Sue Colin would say. So I danced with my fear. It was uneasy, awkward dancing but, as the band was playing, I had no choice. Also, at this time, I had a low self-image. I didn't like the way I looked physically; I felt I was five pounds overweight. Before surgery five extra pounds made me feel voluptuous, zaftig, very womanly; now I felt out of balance. It was one thing to have two full breasts and rounder hips, but it was another thing altogether to have one full breast, heavier hips and full cheeks blossoming from under a crew cut. I hated the way I looked, and I didn't like the way I felt. I didn't like much of anything.

I especially didn't like Saturday mornings — getting up, doing Zuleika's hair for her show finals and being too unwell to go along. I remember standing at the gate waving good-bye, watching Charlie drive off with Zuleika sitting beside him looking beautiful, dressed for the important class she was about to ride in.

I recalled when I took her to the shows, tacked up her horses, rode them before she did, groomed and washed them, did her hair, got her ready, schooled her — everything — and now nothing. My life was becoming narrower. Whenever I tried to do something more, it seemed some little thing would go wrong — the phlebitis, a swelling behind my knee, pains in my ribs and lumps around my incision.

I still meditated once a day, but my patience wore thin. I thought perhaps I would feel better if I lost weight, so I decided to work on my self-image during meditation. First healing meditation, then self-image meditation, seeing myself slimmer, more the way I wanted to look. I imagined my hair longer and everything about my body lean and muscle-toned. I hated losing muscle tone. Maybe I could maintain it mentally. It was worth a try.

By now, almost everything we had at the beach house had been packed up and taken to Bel Air, so this day was one of my last to sit in the king-sized bed looking out at the ocean. I knew I might never again live in a house such as this. I knew we probably would not buy a home on the beach. I was happy with the house we had chosen and was eagerly waiting to hear if our new bid was accepted. I knew nothing could replace the majesty and power of the ocean in your backyard. For five months it had served me well. It had been my companion, my friend and a provider of mental and emotional energy.

In spite of my depressed state, basically deep inside myself I didn't believe I had any cancer left in my body. I was mostly irritated by the fiddling limitations of minor health problems. All the commands to rest and take care of myself tied me down. I was sure a few months down the line I would be my old self, but for now it was goddamned uncomfortable to be so close to the end and yet not at my destination. I could see the light at the end of the tunnel and I was anxious to get there.

I needed a change of pace, so the next day on my way home from Bernard's I decided to pamper myself a little. I pulled into a shopping center where I knew there was a Christine Valmay beauty shop, which specialized in facials, manicures and pedicures. Ah, me, a pedicure — what a luxury. Just what I needed to lift my spirits, a matching set of deep red toenails.

I had my faithful Cassie in the back of the Bronco. I was also baby-sitting my son Valentine's small blond cocker spaniel, Little Joe Cocker, or Leaky Joe, L.J. for short. They were good company, quite devoted to me and to each other.

I had taken them for a walk on the beach earlier and thought they could tolerate a bit of a sit in the Bronco while I indulged my vanity. I lowered the back window to ensure they would have plenty of air, told them to "stay" and went into the shop.

It was a nice, friendly salon. The girls knew me and were pleased to see me. Yes, they said, they could give me a pedicure, a manicure too if I liked. It wasn't a busy day. As I sat with my fingers soaking in a small bowl, chatting with Jane, the manicurist, I felt my tensions easing. Jane knew I was fighting cancer. We had discussed it the last time I was in. She had a good friend who was starting a course of chemotherapy, a young girl with two small children. I had sent her my good wishes and recommended some books and suggested she try meditation. Today, Jane told me the girl was meditating and doing quite well and thanked me for my good wishes.

My fingernails neatly manicured and painted with clear polish, I was having a cup of tea while both feet soaked in a large yellow footbath of soapy water, when all the operators in the shop congregated at the front window looking out onto the car park.

One of the girls said, "I wonder what's going on. There are three policemen surrounding that truck. They've been there for ages."

Another said, "God, they've got their guns out."

"Look at that crowd. What's going on?"

Something made me lazily inquire, "Really? What color truck?"

Back came the answer, "A brown one."

I jumped up, knocking over the water, and ran to the door. My God, it was true. My Bronco was surrounded by curious onlookers, two police cars and three policemen, one of whom had a large shotgun trained on the back of my car.

I bolted from the shop, wet bare feet picking up gravel as I ran.

"What are you doing? What's the matter?"

I was stopped immediately by a stern-faced officer.

"Don't come any closer. If one of those dogs moves, I will have to shoot it."

"Oh, God no! Why?"

"They have been jumping out and attacking people," the officer said.

I looked into the back of the Bronco and there, sitting side by side looking apprehensively wide-eyed, were Cassie and, barely showing over the top of the back, the small blond head of Leaky Joe.

I flung myself in true Perils of Pauline fashion in front of the dogs, arms spread out protectively.

"Oh, please don't shoot! There must be some mistake!

Don't shoot my dogs! Let me put up the window. They won't move! Oh, please!"

I burst into tears. It was awful, right there in front of everybody. Crew-cut and wet-footed, I became hysterical.

Suddenly at my side was Jane, the manicurist. She put her arm around me and said to the cold-looking policeman with the gun, "You don't have to be so mean to her."

He looked meaner and said, "You get away, lady. You're obstructing the law."

Jane stuck to her guns. "No, I won't. This lady is my client. I'm staying with her. What happened anyway?"

A kinder-looking policeman came over to me and said in a concerned way, "Now don't get upset. Calm down."

I said, "I'm sorry. I can't, I'm just so shocked. Who did they attack?"

"That man over there."

Everybody looked. And, oh, my God, looking very embarrassed, carrying a stick, horror of horrors, was a disabled man. I cried even harder. I went to the man.

"I'm so sorry. How awful for you. I'm so, so sorry. Where did they bite you? Which one bit you?"

"Well," he said almost apologetically, "the small one barked at me as I passed your truck. Then the shepherd joined in. Then the small one jumped out the back window, followed by the shepherd. The small one tore my trousers and grazed my skin. I just want to be sure they've had their shots. I'm not hurt. I'm all right. Please don't be so upset."

By now I was so fraught with guilt and so shocked that I was letting it all hang out.

The mean policeman was disappointed we were getting along so well. He pointed his gun at the dogs more menacingly and said he would have to impound my pets. At this I cried so hard my teeth began to chatter. Jane, seeing I was close to losing all control, said, "Shall I call your husband?"

"Yes," I sobbed. "Call Charlie." And I gave her the number.

"This is Charles Bronson's wife," Jane told the cop spitefully and then ran off to the shop to call him.

Oh, God, I thought, that's torn it. I am now either off the hook or in really big trouble. I visualized Charlie getting Jane's call and steaming down the freeway to my rescue. Maybe he'd side with the police and blame me for leaving the window down. I suspected he would.

"Don't call him," I yelled at Jane's retreating back.

Too late. She didn't hear me.

Oh, boy. What next? Through the window Cassie was positively cross-eyed with the concentration of sitting still, which was odd, because usually when she saw me, she at least wagged her tail. L.J., too, realizing their peril, was sitting motionlessly beside her, his large, black eyes earnest and sincere. I couldn't believe it.

"Are you sure they jumped out? Even the little one? How did they jump back? The tailgate is much too high."

No one appeared to know. I wondered briefly whether Cassie had grabbed Leaky Joe by the scruff of the neck and flung him back into the truck. By now it was clear there wasn't going to be a massacre and things were calming down. My sobs subsided. The mean policeman had failed to convince the nice disabled man to press charges and had gone back to the doughnut stand where I was told he spent most of his time.

The nice policeman told me I had to impound the dogs myself for one month. The third officer had succeeded in keeping the crowd back and was now getting them to move on. Shaky and disheveled I sat down on the side of the disabled man's car. We had a little chat.

"I am so sorry. May I buy you some new trousers?"

"No, that's not necessary. They're just old trousers and it's only a little tear. I'm sorry you got so upset."

He was so nice that I started crying again. I felt so bad for him.

"It must have been awful for you, having two dogs jump out and attack you?"

"Not really. I like dogs. It was my stick, you know. I held it up as I squeezed past your truck to get to my car. I think I frightened your dogs. But now it's all over. You say they have had their shots?"

"Oh, yes."

"You know," he said, "I've had a bad week. I've got lots of troubles and terrible arthritis."

"I've got troubles, too," I said in a small voice.

"I'll bet they're not as bad as mine."

I gave him a look and found myself saying, "I've got cancer."

I got the full shock reaction. He looked at the ground for a moment and then looked right back up at me and said, "God, I'm sorry."

We sat together on the side of his car for a few moments longer. Then we wished each other luck. He got into his car and drove away. I watched his car until it left the car park, then I returned to the salon to await my husband.

Phew, I hoped he would be as understanding as the dogs' victim. I waited apprehensively for thirty minutes. Suddenly, there he was, walking through the car park in his own inimitable prowling gait. Oh, God, please don't be angry, Charlie.

I thought I'd make it worth his while. So I ran into his arms, saying, "My hero. Thank you for coming. I was so upset."

Charlie gave me a big hug and looked around in disappointment.

"I knew I'd miss all the action. Where is everybody? Someone called to say the police were going to shoot the dogs."

"Charlie, it's all over. But it was awful while it lasted. L.J. bit a disabled man."

"Good grief!"

"Then Cassie attacked him."

"Oh, no."

"Then the police came and wanted to shoot them. Then I got hysterical and told everyone I had cancer."

Charlie shook his head in disbelief and said in a resigned, patient way, "Where's your car?"

"There." I pointed.

"And the dogs?"

"In the back."

"Your shoes?"

"In the shop."

"Let's get them and go home. Okay?"

"Okay, Charlie, and thank you for coming."

We said good-bye to the girls at Christine Valmay and I followed his car home with my two fugitives from justice sleeping peacefully on the backseat.

This episode necessitated Cassie's going back to Bel Air to be incarcerated in the yard there while she served her time.

No one ever solved the mystery of how Leaky Joe leaped back into the truck.

The next day, Saturday, was two days before Michael was to attempt to give me my seventh chemotherapy. It was also a big day for Zuleika. It was the day of the most coveted honor for twelve-and-under riders, Honor Darkar Medal. She had ridden the day before in the first round of the finals, and Saturday morning I braided her hair and tucked it neatly into her hunt cap. Charlie drove Zuleika to ride in round two. If she made it to the top ten, she would ride that night in a very fancy finals indeed. She had been riding well, but by now she was tired.

Friday had been grueling. Zuleika had spent sixteen hours in many different classes and had had her ups and downs. Basically, though, her downs were much higher than they used to be and her ups, consequently, were also much higher. We had arrived at the show before eight in the morning, and I watched her first round. It was perfect except for one fence that put her scores lower than they normally would have been. I stayed with her until I became too tired and cold. Then Charlie drove me to the Bel Air house, where I climbed into our king-sized bed in the newly decorated bedroom and took an hour's nap.

That gave me strength to return to see Zuleika ride in the Los Angeles County Finals, another big, prestigious event that evening. I knew I couldn't keep it up. I realized staying until ten o'clock Friday night to watch the finals (in which Zuleika finished seventh) would make it impossible for me to be present first thing next morning. I wanted to see it all, but I couldn't, at least not now.

In previous years I had been the one riding and Zuleika, the one waiting. She was always a good companion. She stayed by my side, awaiting my turn. Once, when she was a tiny girl, perhaps six, I was showing in a jumper class. I stood by the rail watching other riders on the course. Zuleika was aware of my concentration and nervousness. She patted my arm and said, "Try to keep yourself together, Mummy, I'm just going over there for a minute." It was as if she were the mother and I the competing child. Now the roles were reversed; what they should be. I was the mother and she was the competing child, and keeping herself together very well.

Back at the beach house, I thought and watched the sea, and I wondered if my depressions were typical of people undergoing this medical ordeal, or if perhaps it was just me. Had I always been this way? Did I customarily have downs? I didn't think so, but at this point I wasn't sure. I truly wished I knew another woman who had survived this trauma, someone with whom I could discuss everything. It would have been nice. I resolved to offer my services in some way to other women. I knew how much it would have meant to me to talk to a woman like myself before surgery, and at various stages along the way. I think only a person in my position could understand and perhaps say, "You're going to make it. It's okay. You're depressed now, but you'll pull out of it. Just wait and see. Everything's going to be fine." I heard those words from others, but it would have been so much more reassuring hearing them from a woman who had survived the ordeal.

31

DENNIS T. JAFFE'S *Healing from Within* has many helpful chapters on meditation. One, "Pathways to Relaxation," features many simple relaxation exercises. I added these to Dr. Simonton's tape on relaxation. Jaffe's book became my bible. I read a little of it each night before going to sleep. Just having it near seemed to relax me. It had answers to questions on how to keep myself healthy, how to avoid stress and how to avoid letting my life-style slip back into its old, unhealthy ways.

Jaffe quotes the *Bhagavad Gita,* a Hindu guide to life and meditation that predates Christ by centuries:

> *The wind turns a ship*
> *From its course upon the waters:*
> *The wandering winds of the senses*
> *Cast man's mind adrift*
> *And turns his better judgment from its courses.*
> *When a man can still his senses*
> *I call him illumined.*

As I read, I remembered certain moments when my mind had been still. They were rare, indeed, but wonderful: certain times when I was riding one of my horses and everything was going well over a course where I was concentrating deeply; in the past, when I was painting; at times when I was running. When I ran, I counted my breaths for some reason. One, two, three, four; one, two, three, four. That seemed to put my mind deep inside my body or, rather, deep inside my head, and when that happened, my mind would be stilled. It's a moment when one centers totally on a single thing, excluding all other thoughts. It's a wonderful feeling of completeness. You are completely alive. Humanist psychologist Abraham Maslow calls these moments "peak experiences." The more peak experiences, Maslow says, the better and more complete life will become. Lawrence LeShan defines meditation as the process of learning to do one thing at a time. He says by concentrating on a single thing, whether it be your breath, your garden or jogging, you will enter not only an altered state of consciousness but also an altered and more positive state of psychology. I would work on living in the moment again.

I worked steadily at my *I Ching Work Book,* tossing the three pennies and reading my Chinese future.

As I turned from Jaffe's wisdom to ponder the *I Ching,* Charlie telephoned to say Zuleika hadn't made the cut and would not be riding in the top ten that evening. She had ridden well, Charlie said, but it just hadn't worked out.

Zuleika took the phone to tell me all about her ride. "Arrow was a good boy, Mom, but he cross-cantered in the corners." She still wanted to attend the black-tie dinner even though she wasn't riding.

I told her she was a very good sport to go, but I would rather not make the long drive into town if she weren't riding. She sounded disappointed. Charlie got on the phone.

"Charlie, I really don't want to go tonight if I don't have to. Darling, would you talk to Zuleika. It's not that I want her to think of me as ill, but I'd like her to realize I do have to spare my energy for the times I really need it. Going out there tonight would be a waste of energy, especially since we're spending next week in Santa Barbara at another show."

He said, "Okay, I'll talk to her."

I knew Zuleika was disappointed, as I was for her, but I suppose it was character building for both of us.

Cassie, back from the pokey, needed some exercise, so I

took her for a walk on the beach. The walk was hard work, much harder than it had been a mere four weeks ago. Although my mind was more calm and in better shape, my body obviously was not. The pain in my right side was nagging and worrisome throughout the walk. I wasn't so concerned about the pain. Pain I could handle. It was what it signified that bothered me. Naturally, I wondered if it were a recurrence of cancer or maybe a blood clot. I wanted to forget these things and ignore the pain. Still and all, I thought to myself, at least one member of the Bronson family females had done all right this weekend. Katrina had taken her driving test for the first time and passed, a cause for great jubilation. I was proud of her and thought how far she had come. Now she would be driving herself. I could hardly believe it. A new teenage driver in the family. I wondered what kind of car to get her.

Cassie and I walked along the sand for thirty minutes. It cleared my mind. Cassie found me very boring, as I suspect everybody did, when I was in a slump. She spent her days sitting on the porch balefully looking at me through the window. But now she was running down the beach full tilt through the waves. She chased gulls into the water as if she were actually going to run atop the surf. With winter coming, many beach houses had a bare, closed-up look. Some were precariously close to the ocean. Owners placed pieces of plywood in the sand to protect their homes from the big surf and storms that occurred at this time of year. There were many more gulls and sandpipers on the beach today, so Cassie had a field day. By the time we returned to the house, she was sandy, wet and out of breath — and I was much refreshed.

It was still early, so I took my ancient Corvette for a spin. The fuel tank gauge was on empty. I hoped I would make it to my favorite Chevron station so I could give her a big drink of leaded super premium. As always, the car lifted my spirits. True, the pain and feeling of pressure against my ribs hadn't disappeared, but since the walk, I felt so much better I didn't care. At least I wasn't morbidly brooding about what it might be. I filled the car and took a little drive. I liked being myself.

I made a mental note to remember that. I had been surrounded by people all week and hadn't enjoyed enough solitude. Perhaps the way to deal with depression was to take a
day alone and do whatever I wanted — meditate, throw I
Ching, walk with Cassie, drive my car. These were nourishing
things, nurturing things, "take care of Jill" things. It might
be good to wallow in depression and then climb out of it.
Yes, the day wasn't turning out too badly after all.

I turned the car in the direction of the house on which we
had bid. It was such a pretty place, half-hidden by its wall. I
tried to imagine it was already mine. I daydreamed about
going through the front door to find pieces of my favorite
furniture in place. This was fun, but a little limited, so I
turned the Corvette around and drove to the barn.

Now my day was complete. I visited with the horses that
hadn't gone to the show. The Connemara, Turtle, showed me
rather a fierce eye. I bet he hadn't been turned out today, so I
went looking for Julio, who had worked at the stable for
nearly ten years. I asked if the horses had been out and he told
me he thought Sue Overholt was coming to take care of
them. I asked him to exercise the stay-at-homes and then
drove home.

Charlie and Zuleika were there. They seemed in good spirits. Zuleika had overcome her disappointment and was already
looking forward to the next day's equestrian challenges. Tony
arrived for dinner holding a bunch of flowers and wearing a
happy, somewhat shy smile. As my stepson embraced me with
a big, warm hug, I felt centered and happy.

The following day I stayed home again while Charlie took
Zuleika back to the show. It was a damp, misty day. It made
me think of England and my childhood. I called my mother
and had a long chat. I also spoke to my father, who enjoyed
the conversation even though he could say no more than "lo,
lo, lo" and, being quite deaf, could hardly hear me. Even so,
the variety of inflections he put into "lo, lo, lo" made conversation of a sort. It was good to hear his voice and to have
some communication with him. When he'd had enough, he

would simply go, leaving me in midsentence. Then it was my mother's turn to talk again. I knew it meant a great deal to her to have someone to talk to. She couldn't really converse with my father. She wished me well for my next chemotherapy. She said she would be thinking of me, then said, "Love you, Jilly. Good-bye."

Alan called. He was thoroughly bored with the movie, and I heard a confused sadness in his voice. Then he casually mentioned there was a sound man on the movie who was making remarks, things like "That one's a little light on his feet." When Alan spoke to the makeup girl, the sound man would ask her, "Who's your girlfriend?" I was outraged. Arsehole! How dare he talk to my friend like that. How dare he do anything to spoil Alan's day. Alan loved my fury. He laughed at my rage and my language.

"Oh, it doesn't matter, honey. The only thing is I have to be careful or it can bring back memories of being a teenager and some of the things that were said to me as I was growing up. That's depressing if I let it get to me."

I told him I loved him, that he was a good person, a good man, and I hated the macho bastard who felt he had the right, on a movie set of all places, to make those remarks. I was furious. Boy! Alan said he would call the following evening after my chemotherapy.

Before throwing the I Ching again, I looked once more at yesterday's message: "The yielding and responsive quality of nature is the focus of time. Nature follows with sensitivity the demands of the season. It reproduces, adapts and evolves itself appropriately. It heals itself when injured and deftly maintains a balanced economy." I read on. One line seemed to sum up what I had been doing the past two days: "The power of this time lies in reacting with a natural response to the myriad things around you, a response in keeping with the laws of nature." By going with my feelings — and not fighting them — by resting, thinking and responding to myself mentally and physically, I had been reacting with a natural response to the myriad things around me.

The message said further: "By maintaining a pose of natural response even in the complex matters of business and politics, you can be assured that you are attuned to your own nature."

Today it all seemed to make sense. "You can begin to rely too much upon your own strength and forget that strength can be perilous when not directed properly." That created a picture of myself butting my head against the wall. "This time is a subtle study in nonaction as a way of attaining real meaning in your life."

That line summed up my attitude toward my illness. I read on. Once more a line leaped out at me. "Within yourself spend time alone in objective thought as you consider the direction of your life. Meditate upon the idea that everything on earth, good and evil, is supported by nature. Strive to broaden your attitude and opinions and view the world with an open mind." I loved the next bit: "Objectivity will keep your natural response pure while it gives you great stamina of character and inner calm in dealing with the outside world." I thought if I were a Victorian lady, I would start sewing a sampler with *Keep Your Natural Response* stitched on it, surrounded by flowers. Of course, if I were a Victorian lady, I probably wouldn't have called Alan's critic an arsehole. I was much better today. All the turgid, murky thoughts were gone. I knew I was compelled to go through last week's depression, but now it was a faint memory. I was refreshed and ready to start once more.

32

MONDAY MORNING — CHEMO DAY. I was still feeling well. I took my first Decadron pill, then got back into bed and snuggled into Charlie for a while with the usual results from good, warm snuggling. This was a nice way to start the day, and I figured that whatever went down, the day had had a good beginning. Zuleika left for Santa Barbara with Sue Overholt. They were going to the big national horse show we had been attending for approximately nine years. We always enjoyed Thanksgiving at the Santa Barbara Biltmore. All the family collected for the traditional dinner. Zuleika couldn't remember Thanksgiving anywhere else.

I told Zuleika I would join her as soon as I felt able. My treatment was scheduled earlier than usual, so Charlie and I left the house at noon. I felt well en route to Michael's office; however, as we drove into the underground parking lot, I experienced the usual sinking feeling. The nausea and lack of equilibrium hit me when I put on the ice helmet. Michelle administered the injection slowly, but we injected the wrong vein, so it was a bit painful. By the time I'd been given all three drugs I felt sick and down. I knew it would be a rough night. I was right. I was sick all night and most of the next day, Tuesday. However, late Tuesday afternoon my body rallied. I decided to make the trip to the Turkey Show the next day.

Wednesday started on an up note. The real estate office

called to say our bid had been accepted. We were definitely buying the house. On the drive to Santa Barbara I chatted happily about the plans for our new home with Charlie. Charlie tried to quell my enthusiasm, saying he didn't want me to be disappointed if something went wrong before escrow closed. But I was too happy to be cooled down.

We sailed into the Biltmore and unpacked. Zuleika and Sue were still at the show grounds, so Charlie and I had time to listen to the Mexican musicians in the lobby while we ate nachos, guacamole and refried beans. I sipped white wine and Charlie enjoyed his usual Campari and soda. In all the years we had been coming to the hotel, we had never done that before. Usually I went straight to the show grounds to ride and care for the horses. And each day thereafter I'd be up at six and leave at seven in time for the first class. I'd remain on the grounds all day, returning to the hotel in the evening dirty, tired and ready only for a shower and room service. This year was different. I had no duties either to myself or Zuleika. Sue Overholt had taken over my role.

The week after each treatment I became depressed, sometimes doomsday depressed, sometimes only a little. But always depressed. This week at Santa Barbara the depression was severe. We drove from the Biltmore to the Earl Warren Show Grounds. Everyone around me looked so healthy and strong. It was as if I were the only one present who was ill. I rode Cadok, feeling like a pariah, imagining everybody was thinking how crummy I looked and that I was not long for this world. It was as if "cancer" were embroidered on the back of my jacket and across my brow. I put it down to the chemotherapy. Michael said when I went off the mood-elevating Decadron pills I plunged into this state of mind. The physical and mental fatigue I endured waging war against chemo's side effects probably had something to do with it also. Chemo number seven didn't leave me so weak as chemo number six, when I had been so depleted that I felt that if I closed my eyes and stopped concentrating I would die. This time I was okay physically. Only my mind was in bad shape.

I determined to get with it and just think thoughts as they came to me. I wandered around the rows of tents housing the horses. The show had a carnival atmosphere. Rock music blared from the grooming stalls. Stables displayed colorful barn logos. There were stalls selling T-shirts, jewelry, food, saddles, bridles, tack, puppies and even miniature ponies. I walked Cadok through the warm-up area, where horses were being exercised on the longe line by Mexican grooms and ridden by trainers, junior riders and amateur show competitors. It was a zoo — a combat zone. Dust flew as horses galloped in every direction. Many were being jumped over two warm-up fences in midarena. There were cries of "Look out!" and "Heads up!" even such barbaric shouts as "Hit him!" I actually heard "Rip his teeth out" from an anonymous female voice. The trainers became deeply involved schooling their students. Although he was an old show campaigner, Cadok spooked from all the action, so I left the confusion of the ring and stood for a while at the rail, watching, remembering and looking for Zuleika.

I had a satisfying conversation with Tommy Lowe, horse trainer and friend. He asked how I was. I said, "God, Tommy, it's tough. This damned thing. I feel so isolated and the chemo is a harsh, rough affair. I don't think I could go through this again if I ever had to. I don't think I'd do it."

Handsome, dashing Tommy looked at me and griped right back, "I wouldn't. I tell you I wouldn't."

I loved it. Here was someone who was letting me gripe and complain and agreeing with me. Wonderful! The conversation was perfect. I complained and he took it and agreed. He listened and did not try to cheer me up. Thank God. I loved it; he was perfect. For a while I didn't feel so alone. I almost felt normal. God bless Tom. Talented, sensitive, with masses of problems of his own, he gave me just the reaction I needed — an honest one. No bullshit here, at least not today.

On Thanksgiving, all the family arrived for dinner at the Biltmore. I ordered guacamole, refried beans, hot sauce and lots of crunchy chips as side dishes. Then just as we were all tucking in before dinner with our predinner drinks, I yelled, "Oh, fuck," thereby shattering my mother image for good and all. The reason for my quaint Victorian profanity: I'd broken a tooth off on a chip. The whole damn tooth just snapped off almost to the gum. This grisly event was painless for some contrary reason, however, and I cheered up and really enjoyed dinner and the family's company.

Scanning my brood's faces possessively, I dove right in and chewed on my stump, enjoying seeing Jason and Tony revert to six- and eight-year-olds, giggling together as they had when they were all small. The boys had all been so close, Paul, Tony, Jason, and Val. I used to call them Bronson's Gorillas as they faced the world together. They could fight and beat on one another, but should an outsider threaten one of the clan, he'd better watch out — the whole gang would come down on him en masse. Suzanne, as the only girl at that time, was teased, protected and loved by all of them equally. It was great to be all together. Zuleika and Katrina sat at the far end of the table, heads together, gossiping and whispering as they eyed Jason's beautiful girlfriend, Rena. I knew they were taking in Rena's stylish black leather skirt, boots and cute tam-o'-shanter with its glittering junk-jewelry pin. Suzanne watched in wry amusement. Thanksgiving was a time when the children became, just that once more, children. It gave me a wonderful sense of continuity.

By Sunday I was almost myself again. And as was my pattern, by Monday I clicked over to normal. My energy was back and nothing could depress me. I'm sure this was a great relief to Charlie. I knew I had been a boring companion for most of the week. I had tried not to burden him with my morbid thoughts of death, dying and cancer recurrences, but I knew I hadn't exactly been Little Mary Sunshine.

33

WE DROVE BACK TO THE Bel Air house and I saw it with new eyes. I'd said good-bye to the beach house on Wednesday when we left for Santa Barbara. Now that was history. My old home was gleaming. The wooden floors and paneling had been refinished and showed their true beauty. The dining room table had been set for dinner and looked lovely. It is an English antique and easily seats twelve. It glittered with silver, crystal, linen serviettes and place mats. The room had pale cream linen walls and a cream, pastel blue and green Oriental rug. Antique paintings hung from crimson ribbons on the walls, silver ornaments shone in the candlelight. I walked in knowing never again in my life would I have such a dining room. A carousel horse stood in the window looking at me. "Will there be room for you in the new house?" I thought. He looked concerned.

My house looked beautiful all over. The bedroom had turned out better than I imagined. I was saying good-bye with love and leaving it looking its best. Sixteen years of living invested here, but now it was time to move on. But it would be difficult to leave such beauty. Charlie was sad. He walked around saying, "You really did a good job decorating, Jill." Then later, "This house is built like a fortress." Then, "I don't know why we have to leave it."

I jumped in hastily, "Twelve bedrooms, Charlie, twelve bedrooms."

Still, we were uneasy and sad at the thought of change. I suggested, "If you love this house so much, why don't we spend one last Christmas here. Let's give the children one last big family Christmas in the house they grew up in."

Charlie was shocked, outraged. "You mean not go to Vermont?"

God, I'd said it. It had been on my mind for months, and now I'd said it. "Yes, not go to Vermont." The thing we were both afraid of for different reasons. Charlie had been looking forward to the holidays in Vermont for months. He couldn't believe I had suggested staying in Los Angeles. I wanted to have my last chemotherapy and stay put. Besides, the house was looking lovely and the children had been reared here. It seemed appropriate we should spend one last Christmas in this house. Charlie's son, Tony, would be able to see both his father and mother on Christmas Day instead of having to choose. I wouldn't have to pack all the gifts and do the myriad necessary things involved in leaving for Vermont for the holidays. I could concentrate on recovering from my final chemo and get on my feet without the pressure of the long trip hanging over me.

Well, the pressure had been building for a long time and Charlie and I had *the big fight.*

Charlie, like most men confronted by a crying woman, was frustrated, which in turn led to resentment at being made to feel these emotions. These feelings got in the way of his being able to express the tenderness that I needed. The fact that I knew he had reservoirs of enormous compassion drove me desperately on like a junkie needing a fix, driving further from me with every outburst the very thing I needed so badly. I accused him of being unsympathetic, knowing that with every word I was digging myself deeper and deeper into a hole.

Charlie raged. I wanted love and understanding and to be held, but it's hard for a man to love and hold a prickly pear. He could not help but wonder how my being a cancer victim would affect the rest of his life and the rest of our life together.

Charlie always knew how to tap into my emotional energy, and I sure knew how to push his buttons. So we ranted and raved, taking it as far as we could or dared, until we had enough. Then we'd rest awhile until one of us thought of something else to bring up and we'd start again. We had both been under such immense strain during the long six months of living with cancer in the family. I felt I had lost so much, and Charlie had just been sitting out the whole thing with me. We needed a good blowout.

We went to bed with the situation unresolved. I had been taught by my mother never to go to sleep on a quarrel. Charlie had taught me many years ago that you certainly *can* sleep after a quarrel. At least he can. I was uneasy and spent most of the night awake and thinking. The next day we picked up where we had left off, but by lunchtime we called a truce and went out to a nice Italian restaurant where Charlie agreed, "Okay, we'll stay. Maybe we can take a ski trip for a few days, so we'll get some snow and skiing in."

We settled down to plan. We asked my brother, John, and his family to spend Christmas with us in Los Angeles, instead of Vermont as they usually did. We would have a big family Christmas with my two nieces, Lindsay and Courtenay, brother John, sister-in-law Sandra, Zuleika, Katrina, Paul, Suzanne, Tony, Jason, Valentine, Charlie and me — a cast of thousands — all together opening our presents. I was exhausted emotionally from the decision and all the arguing, but now everyone seemed quite happy with the new plan.

However, I was nervous, tense and resentful. I didn't like feeling responsible for all the changes in our lives. But at the same time, they hadn't been bad changes for my family, just changes. After all, Vermont wasn't going anywhere. It would still be there next year. I just hoped I would. I needed a slap for thinking that thought. I had been feeling sorry for myself too long, but I didn't slap myself, I slipped into an angry state of mind. Damn it, I didn't want any of this. I wasn't able to sleep at night. I went to bed and slept for two hours and then woke up to stay awake for hours with my mind racing, full of rage.

Then one morning I was leaving for an appointment with Bernard Dowson only to be told by my brother-in-law Dempsey, who works for us as Charlie's right-hand man, that the old Corvette's battery was dead, the Jeep's taillights were out and the turn indicators weren't working. I couldn't contain my anger. My cars had worked fine all summer. While we were in Santa Barbara they were driven to Bel Air for me and now this. I slammed out of the bedroom, down the stairs and out the front door, slamming it hard, risking the stained glass. I took the Rolls-Royce to Bernard's. I was driven and desperate. Everything was unfair. While we were fighting, Charlie said one of his rewards was going to Vermont. Well, where were my rewards? He had his ski trip. What was I getting? I didn't expect anything, only not to have him angry with me. I drove crying on the freeway. Because it was the Rolls I couldn't take Cassie. Charlie didn't like dog hair in the car. I missed her badly. I talked to myself.

"I can't take any more. I must be by myself. I'll stay out all day. I must have my own space. I really want the new house to myself." I knew I really didn't want the new house to myself. I didn't want to lose Zuleika or Katrina or Charlie, but at the moment I really needed to keep talking.

"I need to get rid of a lot of things. I want to give away all my clothes. I'll get some big boxes and do it. I'll give *everything* away, than I'll feel lighter."

I drove on, trying not to cry, wiping tears from my eyes so I could see, thoughts coming thick and fast.

"I want to be by myself for the day. I'll get my hair done. I feel so fat and ugly." More tears. "I miss my breast so much. I want to lose weight. I want to give away all my clothes. I don't want anything. I want to live alone. Charlie's depression over canceling Vermont makes me do things I don't want to do just to end his depression. I don't want to go skiing. I want everyone else to go without me and leave me alone. I feel out of control of my life. I have no choices. I feel so lonely and that's okay as long as I can be alone. I don't want to be with people and lonely at the same time. I'm bitter and angry with everyone. I've always tried to do the right thing; and now when I need people to do the right thing by me, no one wants to do it."

That was unfair; nobody knew what I wanted. But I thought it anyway and raged away at the steering wheel, the windowpane, the freeway and other drivers.

"They will do what I want, but only if I force them. I don't want that. I don't want to have to fight for my life on every level. The main fight is just for life itself. I can't afford to use energy fighting for life's compassion and understanding as well. I need sympathy and nurturing. I don't want to fight for love and sympathy when I'm down. That's when I need nurturing for the strength to go on. I can't afford to use my energy then. I need love then."

I drove and ranted and ranted all the way to Bernard's. There I parked the car, wiped my eyes and went in. I avoided conversation with Betty, Bernard's kind receptionist. I walked straight past her and upstairs to lie on the table. For a whole hour I cried quietly to myself.

When my time was up I left without saying good-bye and drove to the Good Earth restaurant. I ordered lunch and then called Charlie. He must have been in the shower, so I called the other line and asked Dempsey to tell Charlie I was going to stay out all day. After lunch I called Charlie again.

"I'm really upset, Charlie. I feel really up against it. I need time to myself. I'm going to stay out all day. I don't want you to worry. That's why I'm calling."

Charlie sounded hurt and annoyed. "What are you going to do? And what do you mean you don't want me to worry about you?"

"It makes no difference to me if you worry or not, so just be comfortable. Do what you like. My cancer and I are spending the day alone. I'll see you at dinnertime."

I paid my bill, got into the car and drove to Malibu. I was still upset, rebellious and crying at intervals. I went to my hairdresser and asked her if she could wash and trim my hair. She said she could in fifteen minutes, so I called Charlie again. For someone who wanted to be alone, I sure called him a lot. I tried to tell him all my feelings.

He said, "Why are we talking on the phone?"

I started to cry. I said I couldn't talk anymore and hung up. My hairdresser gave me a cup of camomile tea, which calmed me. I had my hair washed and drove home, calm enough not to talk to myself on the drive.

When I got into the house and saw Charlie sitting in the study reading a script, my mood returned. I needed to talk, so I poured out my feelings. I talked and cried.

"It's so hard, Charlie. I'm worried all the time. I think I may die in the next two years or maybe five. I've lost so much. All my hopes and dreams. I hate having one breast, and I keep waiting for the other shoe to drop. I have a burning sensation in my left breast just like I had in my right one before the biopsy. I think it's cancer. I hate the prosthesis. It's not for me; it only works for everybody else to make them feel better when they look at me. That way they don't have to be reminded of what's happening. But it doesn't have that effect on me. All it does is remind me. It's so damn uncomfortable. It's always slipping and out of place. I hate my hair and I hate myself." I cried and cried and cried and cried. Poor Charlie.

He said, "Please come over here and let me hold you."

I was furious. "No, I don't want to be touched. I just want to sit here and cry. If you hold me, it will stop me. You see! Now you've done it, I've stopped now just talking about being held." I had been on a good roll; now I couldn't get it back. Poor Charlie. He couldn't do anything right today so far as I was concerned. "I don't need to be held," I snapped. "I just want to cry."

"But I need it for me," he said.

"Oh, okay," I said ungraciously and went over to the big red leather chair in which he always sat, and curled up on his lap. It felt good. I cried more but not so angrily and very soon I calmed down. Charlie sensed this.

"Would you like some tea?"

I did feel much better. I had released my feelings.

Now I was ensconced comfortably in my own red leather chair, drinking the best, most delicious cup of tea I had tasted for a long time. I was thirsty and dehydrated from all my crying. A wonderful calm came over me. I loved Charlie and told him so. Now all I had to do was get my allergy test for Novocain, get my tooth fixed, get my blood test, get my left breast felt up to get rid of all my cancer worries, get my last chemotherapy, and then I could enjoy Christmas.

34

MY CRAZINESS PASSED AND the next few days I chipped away at my "to do" list. I took the allergy test and was told Novocain could be safely used. My fractured tooth was fixed. I strolled into my surgeon's office unannounced to find the waiting room empty. Dr. Karlan was away, but Dr. Uyeda was there. He examined me carefully and said he could feel nothing wrong.

I told him, "I know I worry about everything, but I think I should. I know I'm a high-risk patient, so I feel I can't afford to ignore anything."

He looked into my eyes for a long time. Then he said, "I know, but you're going to be okay. All right? Hang in there. I guarantee it." Dr. Uyeda put out his hand and shook mine. He continued looking at me steadily. I knew he was trying to help, so I bought it. I was in no mood to fight today.

At home I talked on the telephone with a television scriptwriter, a woman I hadn't spoken to for two years. She was also a cancer victim, fighting leukemia for seven years. She sounded as if she had a cold.

"No," she said. "I'm just fighting this damned leukemia." She didn't have to tell me she'd been crying, but when she heard my voice she picked up immediately. She was happy to talk to me for the first time in such a long while. We brought each other up to date on our lives. Then, inevitably, she asked, "Well, how are you, Jill?"

I paused. It was getting easier for me to say, "Well, I've had six months of chemotherapy." That told her the whole story.

"I'm so sorry, Jill."

"But I'm fine, Allison, really I am. I've only one more treatment. I'm doing holistic healing using the O. Carl Simonton method."

"I know of him," she said.

"And I go to a homeopathic doctor and have treatments on his electromagnetic table." I found myself urging her to go to Bernard Dowson. I explained what he did and how it worked. I ended up saying, "Well, Ally, I believe it won't hurt and maybe it will help."

"Oh, you're just like me," she said. "That's the way I think."

I promised to call Allison again soon and told her to telephone if she needed a good complaining session or sympathy. I said I would do the same. We agreed it was not something one could do too often with one's husband.

I said, "If anyone has any illusions left about catastrophic illness being a romantic situation, as in the movies, forget it. After the first shock, it's business as usual. Right? Life has to go on and, after all, isn't that what it's all about — life going on? Don't you find that in the beginning one hears oneself saying, 'How can he/she/they say/do/behave that way to me? I've got cancer.' Actually, though, I think it's normal behavior that keeps you going."

Allison said, "Yes, it's a good thing to develop a network of friends with whom you can let down once in a while."

She said she was so low recently that she'd gone into the bathroom, looked at all the pills and thought about doing away with herself, then decided it would be "too tacky."

"She's a brave woman" flashed across my mind, fighting all these years. As long as I'd known her, she'd been living under the sword. When I hung up, I felt such compassion and understanding.

I suddenly missed my father and his challenging, indomitable will. Even though conversation was virtually impossible due to his deafness and his aphasia, I made a telephone call and was delighted by my father, who greeted me in full voice, singing — which he could still do, curiously enough — "Poor little dickie birds out on the sea. Poor little dickie birds, oh dear me."

This cracked me up. My father, clever old man, knows he can no longer speak and has been instructed by my mother that when she is out he must never answer the telephone. He can, however, sing lyrics, songs he remembers from before the stroke destroyed his communicative powers.

I said, "Hi, Daddy, how are you?"

My father laughed loudly, happy that it was me and that he wouldn't be in trouble later. He then treated me to "The north wind doth blow and we shall have snow, and what will poor Robin do then, poor thing?"

He paused and I replied, "He'll sit in the barn and keep himself warm."

Then we sang in unison, "And hide his head under his wing — poor thing!"

We both laughed. I said, "Daddy, you're so naughty; you're not supposed to answer the phone but I'm glad you did. How are you feeling?"

A very serious voice said, "Ahhh, lo, lo, lo," in descending tones.

I said, "Now, Daddy, if you're worried about me, you have no reason to. It's not too easy to keep an Ireland down, you know."

"Ahh, hahh," said my father.

Then I asked if he would like to sing again.

His voice brightened as I launched into "Any time you're Lambeth way, any evening, any day, you'll find them all doing the Lambeth Walk."

"Oy," said my father.

"Good-bye," said I.

And he hung up. My father was given to abrupt telephone terminations.

I knew he would enjoy the song. I had taken him only nine

months earlier to see a revival of the musical that first featured it — *Me and My Girl* — and it reminded me of the tragicomedy of errors that had occurred in London on that outing.

I was staying at the Dorchester Hotel with Zuleika and Katrina. We had the beautiful Oliver Messel Suite. I was to be visited by my parents and my mother's sister Edith. I hadn't seen my Auntie Edie, as I called her, in several years and it had been months since I had seen Mummy and Daddy. They were expected at 11 A.M. Dressed in a pink silk skirt and matching sweater, with newly washed hair, looking like Daddy's little girl, I waited for them in the lobby.

I waited until noon. Then beginning to feel self-conscious and a bit wilted, I bought some flowers for my mother and aunt and returned to the suite to wait. My family arrived at twelve-thirty and sat in the lobby for half an hour. The hall porter misinformed my parents that I had gone out. There they sat, waiting expectantly, until Zuleika went down to see if they'd arrived. She came upon them sitting in a rather sad little group listening to a pianist as he entertained the guests. Upstairs I was nervous. What could have happened?

Suddenly, bing-bong, the doorbell. They were here. My aunt and mother bustled in.

"Lo, lo, lo," a gruff masculine voice was saying. "Lo, lo, lo."

There he was, my father, white hair and mustache, a ruddy glowing face, eyes snapping with the excitement of seeing me, sporting a brown tweed jacket, blue shirt, brown silk tie, black slacks and black leather running shoes fastened by strips of Velcro. Gripped in his left hand was a stout wooden walking stick. His right arm lay limply by his side. It was paralyzed. Maybe he couldn't speak words anymore, but by God he made his presence felt.

He looked at me, his daughter, his eyes boring holes into my face. I felt the question and I gave the answer.

"I'm well, Daddy. Really fine. How are you?"

He gave a triumphant laugh, head thrown back. The laugh was aimed at the gods. His eyes were sparkling.

"He's been geared up for this visit ever since he heard you were coming to England," said my mother.

"Yush," said my father. He didn't take his eyes off me. I helped him get seated in one of the big comfortable green velvet armchairs in the suite. Zuleika and Katrina told my mother and aunt about the things they had been doing in London. The excitement in the room mounted.

"It's good to see you looking so well," whispered Auntie Edie. "Where's Charlie?"

"He's working today. He won't be home until this evening."

My father just sat there beaming, the patriarch looking around at the womenfolk, his daughter and granddaughters, sister-in-law and wife.

"Lo, lo, lo," he said, pointing to his jacket.

"Very smart, Daddy."

"John bought it for him last summer," my mother told me.

"Lo, lo, lo." This time the right hand flipped his tie into the air.

"Yes, Daddy, I remember; it's an old one of Charlie's. You look so smart. You're still a handsome old devil."

"Yush," said Daddy.

We were going to the matinee performance of a revival of the 1937 musical *Me and My Girl*. It started at 3 P.M. "You should enjoy the show. You'll know all the songs, Daddy," I said.

My mother looked sharply at my father. "Jack! Where's your hearing aid?"

"Lo, lo, lo?"

"Your hearing aid." She raised her voice. "Oh, you forgot to put it on. Now you won't hear the music properly."

"Don't worry, Mummy, I've got seats right down front. He will hear and see everything really well. Let's order a light lunch before we go."

But she wasn't finished. "Jack! Where are your glasses?"

"Lo, lo?" This time the triumph was fading in his eyes.

He'd forgotten them too. He had failed — hearing aid and glasses.

Oh, well, not to worry. We did have seats down front. Soon everyone piled into the limousine. Daddy sat in front with the driver, happily looking at the sights. He had been born and raised in London. It was his town. He knew every stick and stone. Soon he began to direct the driver in "lo, lo" as to the quickest route to the theater. In spite of this, or maybe because of it, we arrived at the theater with ten minutes to spare. I led my little band in. The lobby was full of old people, a sea of white, fluffy heads eagerly anticipating the show.

Disaster struck again. There was a mix-up with my tickets. I wasn't booked for the matinee performance. Someone else had the six seats in third row center. I couldn't believe it. My parents' wonderful afternoon was being ruined.

I was angry. I lost my sweet image in one word. "Oh, shit." I wanted to see the manager. He arrived full of unconcerned concern. It was a simple mistake and there was nothing he could do. My tickets said matinee as I requested, but someone — and naturally no one knew who — had written "evening performance" at the box office. My carefully chosen seats were gone. I stood fuming, watching my family confused and anxious, aware of my discomfort. They knew something was amiss. My "Oh, shit" had resounded rather well through the foyer. Finally I was given an apology, a box of chocolates and six tickets in the back row off to the side. Daddy couldn't see without his glasses, nor hear too well without his hearing aid, but at least he had an aisle seat in which to jut his cane.

The show commenced. I was still so angry I could hardly sit still. Daddy yawned once or twice as the show passed dimly before his eyes. My mother, bless her soul, made the most of it, eating the chocolates and laughing at the old jokes.

"Want an aperitif?" says the butler to the cockney.

"No fanks, I've got my own," was the reply.

Mummy laughed in appreciation. My father didn't hear.

Oh, Daddy, I wanted you to enjoy your day — I was communicating with him telepathically. I was still too upset to relax. I was stiff across my shoulders and my head was aching. Suddenly it happened. The orchestra struck up "The Lambeth Walk," the song of Daddy's youth, the song of London: "Any time you're Lambeth way, any evening, any day, you'll find them all doing the Lambeth Walk. Oy!"

Daddy straightened in his seat, his whole body stiff with recognition. The orchestra was going full throttle now. From the back of the theater the cast, dressed as cockney costermongers, came running past my father, singing at the top of their lungs, "You'll find them all doing the Lambeth Walk."

"Oy," one of them shouted at him.

I looked at Daddy. Tears were spouting from his eyes, gushing down his cheeks. "Oy," he said.

A sob escaped him as he joined in. "Doing the Lambeth Walk," he sang.

My heart was bursting, my throat constricted. I tried to sing with him, but every time I tried I came too dangerously close to outright crying. I put my arm around his shoulders and patted him in time with the music. I could hear my mother and auntie singing on my right. But I was tied in close to Daddy. We were doing the Lambeth Walk.

I looked at the telephone and said silently to him, "Thank you, Daddy. You inspired me. You gave me the courage to keep on going. I love you."

Somewhere in England I could almost hear his voice joining mine — "Doing the Lambeth Walk. Oy!"

35

CHRISTMAS WAS FAST approaching. As we were not going to Vermont and as I told everyone I was not buying as many gifts this year, I reduced pressure on myself. Charlie was resigned and I felt comfortable about it. I knew how much he looked forward to his weeks' skiing, and I felt sad about taking away his white Christmas. The Colorado ski trip would help.

One night in bed, I asked Charlie if he ever was scared I would die, that I would get cancer again. He said, "Of course, but I prefer to be optimistic and hopeful. There's hardly a minute of every day that I don't think of you and your situation."

It was strange how *optimistic* and *hopeful* struck chords of fear in my gut. He also said, "If I thought you weren't going to make it, how could I live with you every day? I'd just be waiting for you to die."

God, I was shaken hearing Charlie speak like that. I had thought I wanted Charlie to go through it all with me, blow by blow, oozing compassion, sympathy and understanding, but, in fact, the reverse was true. Now I realized I wanted this one relationship to stay the same — normal. I didn't want to see Charlie scared or overly sympathetic. Deep inside me, at the root of my convictions, I knew that while my relationship with my husband remained normal — not too much sympathy for me or for himself — I was going to be all right.

When Charlie came close to being what I had thought I wanted — very *Terms of Endearment,* or *Love Story* — and demonstrated, even unbeknown to himself, fear for my future, it scared me. I had learned my lesson. I wanted Charlie to treat me the way he always had, to yell when I was late for dinner, to tell me off when I complained too much, to fight with me, to criticize, to sometimes bully me and, above all, to love me.

Charlie triggered my survival energy. No more Mr. Nice Guy, Charlie, please! I decided to leave my husband alone to be himself and stop trying to educate him on how to behave with a wife who had cancer. My loving, tough, gruff, quiet, loner husband showed me in so many ways that he loved me. Why had I felt I needed demonstrations of dementia and breast-beating? Well, I know now I couldn't have taken them. I was a flowering cactus, not a hothouse plant, after all.

I had a bad cold the next few days, so I was ostracized from the family and moved into my dressing room. I slept and took meals there to avoid contaminating the rest of the house. I spent three days cooped up, writing, reading and meditating — actually having a rather nice time. By the fourth day, I was feeling better; no more sneezing, and nose-blowing was cut to a minimum. I thought I might get up, but as my energy level was still low, I merely tidied my antique English four-poster and returned to bed with a cup of camomile tea. I popped a Jackie Wilson tape into the player. "You'd better stop yeah-eh-eh-eh-eh leading me around." I joined in with gusto while sipping my tea and looked around my lovely dressing room.

I had created it for myself as a haven, a place to come and dream and to create in its privacy romantic fantasies. When I was depressed, I saw myself in a designer evening gown, sparkling with jewels and moving in a drift of expensive perfume. But now, as I sat in bed looking around, wearing an old flannel nightgown, it was as if the room belonged to someone else. I was only borrowing it. I studied the many possessions the room held, and I couldn't believe they were all mine. In the mirror across the room, I didn't make a romantic figure.

I looked at all my tools for creating illusions: the scarf twinkling with sequins draped over my blond wig on top of a long, narrow antique tallboy embossed with gold. The wig and the scarf summed up the image of a romantc night of dancing, music, wine and laughter; witty, flirtatious conversations with elegantly dressed, suave gentlemen; or perhaps a moonlit ride in an open-top car, a white one, with new-smelling leather and deep, comfortable seats, the sequined scarf blowing lightly in the balmy night air.

It was a room of dreams all right. A blue horse-show ribbon hung suspended from an old silver chain-mail evening purse. Two dreams there. A successful day at the horse show followed by an evening at the ball. There were six tiny painted portraits of ladies in powdered wigs and evening gowns. They were very old and quite beautifully framed. I had bought them in Madrid many years ago. Now they sat on the mantelpiece as if they were my ancestors. I had created quite an atmosphere in which to dress myself. The room fairly reeked of money tastefully spent, liberally spent — all for me — to create the illusion of a fairy princess about to go to a ball.

Well, well, well, I thought as I looked around. You had it all. It's all here to prove it. All your props and devices are still here, exposed. Or in drawers or closets, a lot of them hidden and forgotten, but all of them here. I wondered what I was going to do with them — all the baubles, bangles and beads. I no longer thought I wanted to create an illusion or, to be more honest, the core of me had received a bigger blow than I had at first acknowledged. It was hard to bully a decent fantasy into shape incorporating a one-breasted woman. I had tried.

The beautiful blond woman with her delicate bone structure, long legs and tiny waist danced in the moonlight, shimmering in white chiffon, the scent of camellias wafting from her hair. The dress floated around her as she moved; her partner held her close, feeling the warmth of her body. As they moved to the music, he murmured, "I love you, my dearest, will you be mine?"

She pressed her prosthesis against him. "Oh, yes, Duke, yes," she uttered. Uh-hum.

Well, maybe I'd try the mature, sensual woman fantasy. She oozed into the room, a full-bodied man's woman, sparkling red silk flowing over her perfumed smooth skin, rippling over her perfect undulating hips and dripping over her breast and well-fitted prosthesis. Oh, oh. I wondered how Harold Robbins would handle it.

There was a knock on the door. Lunch interrupted my thoughts, and just in time, too. I liked myself as I was, stripped of all illusions. I surveyed the room. I've got all this stuff — the stuff dreams are made of — but I don't need it anymore.

36

I TALKED TO WILLIE GAYLE, the cancer victim and wife of the actor who had made friends with Alan on location in New England. Willie was in the hospital recovering from surgery. She said her friends came to the hospital, her husband brought the baby, and they were all very close to her before she had surgery. She really thought she would lose her life. But when she returned from surgery, the doctor was very high, saying he'd got most of it. It wasn't the primary cancer that caused this new tumor. It was a whole new tumor the size of a cantaloupe, and he'd removed all but a few small nodules that had entered her uterus, requiring removal of her uterus

I talked to Willie about O. Carl Simonton and asked her to find a copy of *Getting Well Again* and to record the meditations. I suggested she buy Dennis Jaffe's *Healing from Within* as well. When I heard fatigue creep into Willie's voice, I told her to call me anytime. Hang in there, Willie girl. Keep up the good work.

Like me, Willie was fortunate. Her sister was a nurse and had flown in to take care of her baby, and she had many supportive, close friends. She had a cot in her hospital room, where family members took turns spending the night. I was happy for her. I knew how important it was to have that sort of support in time of crisis. I knew I'd been wrong to expect Charlie to support me completely while he was reeling from the impact of having a critically ill wife. I knew Willie's husband must be going through the same thing, and I was glad she had other friends around to help her, and in so doing, help him.

The next day I visited Michael for my blood test. This time, instead of his usual pinprick, he took a considerable amount of blood for more comprehensive testing. He said a complete blood count would be taken to see if there were any malignancies in my system. I had had the same test before surgery and it came back negative, so not all tumors could be detected through the bloodstream. Nevertheless, it would be better to have the test negative than positive, that was for sure. Michael was also going to do cholesterol, blood sugar, kidney and liver tests.

Chemotherapy — a lifesaver. I was grateful it was around and that medical science discovered it in time for me. I loved my life, even with all that had happened. I wanted to stick around. I felt as if I had jumped feetfirst into a deep, black well full of water, going down, down, down. Then, touching bottom, I bounded off and started the trip back up, up, up. I was certain I would break the surface sometime soon after the final treatment.

My body was shaping up not too badly, I thought. The phlebitis had been gone for some two weeks. Although I hadn't started exercising for fear the earlier thrombosis that had occurred after my strenuous exercise on the beach would return, I felt stronger and more secure. After my final chemotherapy, I planned to resume my exercise regime, starting with walks, building up to jogging, stretching, and maybe I'd go back to Jane Fonda's aerobics class. But this was all the future. For now, I must tie up loose ends.

King Zimmerman, Alan's friend, came to decorate the house for Christmas for me. What a dear, sweet man he was. Even Cassie had to admit to a certain affection for him. King literally decked the halls with wreaths and garlands, which he trimmed with real fruit and silk ribbons. The house smelled wonderfully of pine. Charlie had been in charge of buying the

Christmas tree. It was always his job; he liked doing it. In Vermont, he took the snowmobile and chopped down a tree and hauled it back. This year, Charlie bought an eleven-foot fat beauty. With Christmas music playing, he happily strung lights and hung balls while I wrapped a few last-minute gifts and King decorated the wreaths. Charlie was so happy. He truly loved Christmas.

As a child the only gift he ever received was a cellophane-wrapped popcorn ball that the mining town's company store gave to each child in the family. These were hung on the family Christmas tree. Perhaps that was why our tree always gave Charlie so much pleasure. I watched him climb the ladder, painstakingly winding tinsel garlands around the tree, completely absorbed in his job, singing once in a while in his funny, slightly off-tune voice. Charlie Buchinsky, the little boy who once had such belief and faith in Santa Claus that he hung up his little black sock for Santa in a house that was too poor to fill it or even to notice that he did it. In the morning when he got up eagerly to see what Santa had brought for him, it was empty.

It saddened me when Charlie told me the story many years ago. It also gave me greater insight into this man I was married to, a man who found it hard to trust or believe in people. The only person he completely trusted was himself. I could imagine how it must have shaken his beliefs to have his wife become ill with cancer just when it seemed everything was going so well in his life. I sat there wrapping one of the crystals I was giving my son Valentine, watching Charlie and remembering our many Christmases.

My mind drifted back to Christmas when my children were young. On one particular Vermont Christmas, after the children were in bed, I stuffed the stockings and enjoyed a glass of champagne with Charlie in the cozy kitchen, looking out at the largest snowflakes I had ever seen. The snow fell silently all night. It was the perfect picture-postcard Christmas scene with the icicles hanging heavily on the many fir trees surrounding the house. The next day the children made a huge snowman on the front lawn, tying a red scarf around his neck and putting one of Charlie's ski hats on its head. Zuleika was perhaps only three. Everyone was riding around the property on snowmobiles. She wanted to be included, so Charlie tied her small sled to the back of his Snowcat and towed her, lying red-faced on her belly, tightly holding on as she brought up the rear of the excited procession of speeding sleds.

With all my memories, the one I savored and held closest this evening was of a Christmas early in our marriage when I filled one of Charlie's black socks, carefully wrapping a Swiss Army knife, some hard candy, a bottle of his favorite cologne, a bag of gold-wrapped chocolate coins, a small flashlight, a caramel apple and gold and sapphire cufflinks, five ballpoint pens and various other things I thought the child in Charlie would enjoy, and hung it on the mantelpiece in our Vermont bedroom for him to find in the morning. I attached a note: "To Charlie Buchinsky, from Santa. Sorry for the year I forgot." There was no big demonstration from Charlie when he found it. He just took his stocking down and didn't undo it until the end of the day, after all the gifts under the tree had been distributed and each had been unwrapped. The boys were still little children and the house was a noisy, exciting place indeed on Christmas morning. The boys and Suzanne all had their stockings at the foot of their beds, and our day flew by ankle-deep in wrapping paper, ribbons and excited children. In the quiet of the evening, sitting in his special, deep red velvet chair, privately and almost secretively, he opened his stocking, saying nothing, no one to see. Charlie Buchinsky finally got his stocking filled.

Now, I reflected on what sort of Christmas it would have been for my family if I hadn't gone for my breast checkup last June. There was a strong possibility I would not be sharing this moment with them. I found it difficult to believe.

The tree became a work of art. I enjoyed the evening, sipping red wine, feeling warm and nostalgic. The next day's chemotherapy was far from my mind as I watched Charlie and King completely absorbed in their tasks. This night I felt immortal.

37

THURSDAY, THE THIRTEENTH of December. As we drove to Michael's office, I didn't feel especially different, not elated certainly, that this was to be my last chemotherapy. I was a bit numb. Maybe it was the red wine from the night before. Michael came in with the results of my blood test.

"Everything is fine, Jill. The cancer test came back negative. Even though some cancers don't excrete into the bloodstream and therefore don't register, it is not a useless test. We're not looking for the primary cause of your cancer, but maybe a secondary offshoot and it seems that you're clear. Your blood sugar is good, your cholesterol is low, your liver and kidneys are fine." Well, that was good news, a really fine Christmas present. Thank you, Michael.

The treatment got off to a shaky start. Michelle couldn't get a vein. The needle kept slipping out. Finally, I suggested an alternate vein. It worked.

At one point, while I was whimpering and whining, my right hand covering my eyes to avoid watching the dreaded injection, I said haltingly, "Michelle, you may have noticed that I have a very acute . . . a very acute imagination." That sent Charlie and Michelle into peals of laughter. Michael said he would see me in two months. I made the appointment, wished all the girls in Michael's office (especially Michelle) Happy Holidays, Happy Christmas, blew Michael a kiss and went home.

I can't say if the final treatment was worse than the other seven. But it was, significantly, the last.

I was in pretty good spirits. King was sitting in the kitchen with my secretary, Sue. I joined them for a friendly glass of wine and some good conversation. So far, so good. No nausea yet. I just felt a bit squishy inside. Later that night I did feel ill, so I slept in the dressing room again. That way, I could get up and move freely without disturbing Charlie. I didn't want to disturb anyone with my problems. I wanted to handle it gracefully this time.

The following day I did feel off-color, and remained in bed writing Christmas cards and gift tags while my smug little Siamese cat, Polar, purred at the foot of the bed. I was sick all day, but toward evening the nausea passed and I was left fatigued and with a vague sense of unease. I still couldn't quite believe I had had six months of chemotherapy and, contrary to expectations, I had never lost my appetite. In fact, in the past two months I had eaten more than I had since I was last pregnant. I learned that a hearty appetite is not uncommon among people taking chemotherapy and that most women and men add an average of ten pounds. Two popular myths were dispelled: one, that you lose weight and become tragically thin while taking chemotherapy, and, two, that your husband and family will pull you through. You will be supported, but it won't ever be enough. A network of close friends is necessary to help with the difficult days.

It's too threatening for close loved ones to be submitted to your every emotion, too claustrophobic. Support from outside the home keeps personal relationships in better shape and alleviates some of the horrendous stress placed on the victim's family. It's difficult to watch someone you love suffer, and it's hard to listen to a blow-by-blow account of the bad spells. It can be corrosive. As long as all the toxic energy gets a chance to be moved out of one's head, that's all that matters. It's a shame you can't just talk to the wall and get rid of it, but there has to be a receiver. You have to talk out your horrible, bad feelings. Somebody has to receive them, or at least appear to. The right therapist or the right friend is vital.

I don't mean to underestimate how much love and support I received from my husband and children, but it was simply that I needed more than even they could give. I was much too needy at times. No one person could have ever been everything to me. The most important person is the self — to learn to live with your own feelings and not to insist the person closest to you fully understand.

The chemotherapy over, I was faced with picking up my life again — no more excuses, no more weekly trips to the doctor. I was on my own with what I had left, what I had lost and what I had gained. I continued my visits to Sue Colin, although less regularly during the holiday season. I had no ups and downs at this point. During one particular visit I was calm and level. I told Sue my whole body felt immersed in pure crystal water. All was going well.

I saw Bernard Dowson and found him in a state of high excitement. He had invented a new electromagnetic shooter. He said he would shoot a high-intensity magnetic wave into my body, similar to the table but much, much stronger. He ran it over my body, at times focusing on my liver. He said he wanted to clean out my liver and remove all the dead cells from my body. As he applied the treatment, I experienced a deeper relaxation than I'd known at any other time.

Next, I called my hairdresser, Zoren, who hadn't done my hair since before my illness. He came to the house and solemnly trimmed and shaped my inch-locks. It was good for morale just to have Zoren in my life again. I became more my old self. The next morning I stripped off all my clothes and exercised in my dressing room, naked except for my bikini underpants, and analytically watched myself exercise. I thought my body didn't look bad. The one breast was rather nice; the other side, well, it certainly reminded me of my pre-pubescent years when I had a flat chest. I could feel my ribs with my fingers in a place where I hadn't felt them for years. I did leg lifts and stretches and felt much better. As I watched myself in the mirror, I resolved to be kinder to my body, more forgiving; I was going to get back in shape — but gently.

Since my illness, I no longer was in competition with anyone or anything. I would work with what I had now, not what I would try to become or what I had once been. I was grateful for the experience I had been through. God knows I did not want ever to go through it again, but I would not have missed it in spite of everything. The thought of ever having to face surgery again frightened me. It made me sick. But at the same time, I was amazed it actually had not been so bad. I had received so many gifts in the past six months that it was actually worth it — it really was. The pain, the fear, the loss all contributed to an increased self-awareness. I'd learned so much, things that would never have been possible under other circumstances. I saw everything so differently now. I was even grateful for my scar. I watched myself exercising, studying by body and thinking about the last six months, and also about the future.

"It's not so bad, Jill," I said to myself. "I'm grateful and proud. It's really not so bad. I've made it. I've made it through the last six months. Yea, me."

38

THE NEXT DAY I HAD A SURPRISE visitor. Paul called to say his father was in town from New York and would like to visit me before he left again the next day.

I said, "Of course. I'd love it. Invite him over for dinner."

I told Charlie, who said, "I've got plans to play golf with Valentine tomorrow. Maybe David would like to come along and play with us."

It was arranged. David is an excellent golfer; Charlie had only recently taken up the game. It gave him great pleasure. So David, Valentine, Paul and Charlie would play golf in the afternoon. Afterward we would all have dinner together at home. I invited my friend Susie Dotan, who confided that she had always had a crush on David when he was in "The Man from U.N.C.L.E.," and King Zimmerman. I opened a bottle of Marqués de Riscal, remembering that David and I were almost the first to discover it in California, then planned a meal I knew he would enjoy.

In blue jeans, a pretty pale pink angora sweater and my customary black ballet shoes as house slippers, a habit left over from my dancing days, I was in the large wood-beamed sitting room with King, Susie and Charlie. Charlie was telling me how much he and David had enjoyed their golf, when I saw the front door open and two figures enter. I recognized David and Valentine. I stood up, hurrying toward the entryway. David was smiling with his arms outstretched. We held each other for a long time. I hadn't seen him for about four years. We broke apart. David looked down at my feet.

"Still wearing the same shoes? Can't Charlie afford to buy you new ones?"

I laughed, happy that he remembered.

"How are you, David? You look just the same."

"Oh, I'm fine. But how are you?"

"I've had a bit of a rough time, it's true. But I'm all right now."

We walked together into the sitting room, his arm still around me.

"I can feel your ribs," he said.

"Yes? Well, maybe you can. But I'm fattening up now."

I introduced David to King and Susie. Drinks were served and I had the pleasure of watching past and present happily enjoying each other's company. Charlie and David chatted about their day's golf.

David related how the girl who sold golf balls at the club had recognized him and remarked in a cozy, gossipy way, "That's Charles Bronson, isn't it? Didn't you used to be married to his wife?"

David had said wryly, "Yes, as a matter of fact I did."

David smelled the familiar aroma of Indian curry for dinner. He turned to King and said with his head on one side, giving one of his intimate smiles, "When we divorced the only things this lady wanted from me were the children and my curry recipe."

In reply I said, "David, that's not true. I've always wanted your friendship and there's something I've been saving for you all these years."

I moved to a table and picked up a heavy silver serving tray and plopped it into his lap. David looked at it with recognition, "My silver tray."

He told the assembled company that when we were under contract to the Rank Organization every Christmas all the contract artists received a present.

I broke in and said, "We had just been married and were

living in an almost unfurnished apartment. We had so little. Not much more than a bed and a chair. At Christmas we both got these trays. We didn't know whether to use them as sleds or to sell them. This one is yours, David."

David said, "Thank you. I hope it fits in my suitcase."

Dinner was served and we moved into the dining room. Charlie was seated at the head of the table, and I, to soften the stiff formality, sat on his left.

David said to King, who was seated on Charlie's right, "Excuse me, King, may I sit there so I can talk to this lady. I so seldom have the chance."

He took King's place opposite me. Now Zuleika, Valentine, Katrina, Paul, Jason and Susie dispersed themselves around the formally set table. I enjoyed myself, sparkling and flirting, feeling the oppressive months slip away. I was very happy to see David. Happy to have my family and friends together. The evening passed quickly. I could see Zuleika and Katrina were fascinated by my first husband. And Susie confided she still found him most charming and attractive. Charlie obviously enjoyed his company. And as for me, it was like being with a much-loved family member, one who spoke the same language in the same accent. It was so good to see him. A lot of water had passed under the bridge and with it had flowed all traces of bitterness. We were finally free of all hurts. Only our love and friendship remained.

After dinner, when David was leaving, we once again embraced. As we did, I felt the circle was completed. It had taken twenty years, but we had come back to a pure, loving friendship that I knew would last for the rest of our lives. I was moved and grateful that I had lived to experience that healing embrace. What wonderful rewards time can bring.

A few days later John and his family arrived. My tall, handsome brother with his quick wit and generous personality, his wife, Sandra, attractive and elegant, my two nieces, Lindsay, fifteen, and Courtenay, ten. Sweet, sensitive Lindsay with her mother's down-to-earth side and her father's sense of humor, and blond scallywag Courtenay, who I suspect inherited her father's intelligence and business sense, combined with a little womanly bustling quality. An endearing child.

I was at my desk at the top of the stairs when they arrived and I heard the shrieks and laughs and oohs and aahs from Katrina, Zuleika, Lindsay and Courtenay as they greeted one another. This racket played in counterpoint to the masculine sounds that Valentine and John made as they said hello and asked each other the usual greeting-type questions. Here it was again — it was really here — Christmas. We'd gone through another year, and there was to be another large family Christmas, a gathering of the clan under the hospitable roof of the Bel Air house.

The holidays had started. John hadn't been in the house thirty minutes when Charlie grabbed him and the two of them took off on a shopping expedition. Sandra and I knew we'd lost the men for the rest of the day, so we decided to have a tea party. The doorbell rang and it was King Zimmerman.

"Come in, King. We're going to make mango tea, go into the sitting room, look at the tree and have some conversation."

The doorbell rang again. It was my friend Mark with a handsome young Italian named Ciro. Mark came bearing the best shortbread cookies anyone had ever tasted. He'd made them and a large coffee cake. This completed our tea party.

The children came in and hovered around, listening to the grown-ups. I was grateful to be there, so full of warmth and happiness.

Ciro said he liked my hair. "I really like the length. It's so stylish."

I smiled my thanks and thought to myself, "Oh, God, I got a compliment, the first since June second or before." My first Christmas gift — a compliment from a young Italian, a compliment on my hair, of all things.

The afternoon flew by. When John and Charlie returned I

put more hot water in the teapot. Then John and Charlie began their ritual pool game in the area adjoining the sitting room. I could hear the click of pool balls and their shouts and chortles, soon joined by those of the boys Valentine, Jason and Tony. It was a nice atmosphere. Nothing could ever happen to me again, not while I was surrounded by all this warmth and family cheer.

The next day I took John to see Bernard. I wanted him to use the electromagnetic shooter on John to see if it would improve the condition of a tumor in his ear. Bernard used the shooter on me and then it was my brother's turn. John was with Bernard a long time. I hoped for so much. I wanted the treatment to cure John without surgery. Interestingly enough, I found myself in Alan's position, putting all my faith in Bernard and his treatment and believing that if John cooperated, all would be well. I believed in Bernard more for John than I had for myself.

John came downstairs with a calm look on his face and three dropper bottles of the electrically charged water. I made three appointments for John for the following week. I think John's philosophy was "It can't hurt and it probably will help." I noticed he immediately started taking his drops, so he had a little more faith than he admitted. Wouldn't it be wonderful, I thought, if when John returns to Toronto, they tell him his tumor is decreasing.

The next day John, Charlie, Sandra and I went to lunch while Paul took the girls to the Magic Mountain amusement park in the Santa Clarita valley, some thirty miles distant. We had a riotous lunch at Hamburger Hamlet with much full-bodied laughter.

Charlie said, "If you all knew what I was thinking, you'd die."

"In a manner of speaking," my brother added hastily. "What is it?"

"I can't tell you."

"Oh, do tell us," said Sandra, "do tell us."

"No, you're not strong enough to take it — maybe John is, but you and Jill aren't."

Charlie played his game for a while and then announced, "Do you realize the entire Bronson and Ireland families are going on one plane to Aspen for New Year's? There's only one member not going and that's Jason. [Jason had broken his hand and was unable to ski.] Do you know if the plane goes down, Jason will inherit everything?"

"Oh, my God." We all burst out laughing. "That was your big thing?" I asked.

"Jason and Sandra's mother will inherit everything," he said again with a malicious look at John. John burst out laughing.

So did Sandra. "My mother and Jason. It's a funny thought."

I wasn't sure I liked the turn of the conversation. I wasn't even going to ski.

"If it's all the same to everyone, I think I'll stay home with Jason and inherit," I said. On this note, we parted company. Sandra and I kissed our spouses good-bye and watched them set off to do more shopping. Sandra and I hopped gaily into the car and off to — where else? — Neiman-Marcus, or "Needless Markup," as we in the family liked to call it.

It was a full day for me, the longest and fullest since before my illness, but I was energized and enjoying myself. Our mission: to buy last-minute gifts for our Christmas guests — King, my friends Marcia Borie, Kathy Kuzner and Sue Overholt. The others would all be family.

Christmas was only two days away. Sandra and I arrived home just in time for dinner. The back of the small sports car was jammed with packages and paper bags. A new leather jacket for Zuleika (not on the shopping list, but irresistible), a big bottle of Cartier scent for Jason, some Giorgio bath stuff and perfume for Suzanne.

All I wanted for Christmas was a box of Godiva chocolates and a couple of good novels, light reading for a change, and some perfume — and all my senses would be satisfied. I would be in hog heaven, as Alan would say. I knew I shouldn't eat chocolates, and every time I mentioned chocolates to Charlie, he'd say in a stern voice, "Jill!"

But I did hope somebody would break down and bring me some.

39

ON DECEMBER 23 I DEVELOPED a bad head cold. The shopping spree and morning exercises in the nude must have run me down. I knew I had become tired but I was so excited I had kept going. Now I was paying for it. The eve of Christmas Eve Day I was back in my dressing room bed, resigned. Charlie, John and Sandra went shopping again. I had made four huge stockings, one for each of the girls, stuffing them for weeks, buying little things here and there whenever I could. Now they were cornucopias of riches. There were purses and perfumes and chocolates and jewelry — the wonderful, mad, crazy junk jewelry that all the girls loved — bracelets, necklaces and earrings. Then there were beautiful crystals I'd found during the last four months, hand-holding crystals and pendant crystals to wear. Each child received one I'd especially picked for her.

Lindsay's was a glittering pendant with an amethyst. I hung it on a lavender silk ribbon. It was just right for her. Zuleika's was an amethyst as was Katrina's, whose crystal had a pearl at the tip. Courtenay's was an amethyst, too. They were all unusual and quite exceptional. Last-minute shopping produced a denim Guess jacket for Courtenay, who, I'd recently learned from Sandra, dearly wanted one. She had only wanted two things for Christmas — a Swatch watch, which Charlie and I had already found, wrapped and stuffed way down in her stocking, and the Guess jacket. Courtenay would be happy.

Zuleika hadn't asked for anything for Christmas except a fluorescent pink organizer for school. I, of course, bought her that. But, boy, was she going to get a mound of other stuff for Christmas she may not have wanted, but I was pleased to give her. And now I added the leather jacket. Charlie and I loved our child so dearly that nothing was ever too much or too good for her. This didn't make Zuleika spoiled or greedy. In fact, the reverse was true. Zuleika never asked for anything, never coveted anything. I could take her into any store and she'd never say, "Can I have this, please, please?" If she asked for something and I said no, that was the end of it, with good humor. Perhaps there had been so many yeses in her life, Zuleika willingly accepted the nos. The result was a relaxed, happy human being. Zuleika gave us tremendous pleasure.

The girls' stockings were an accomplishment. Four red, green and white gaily striped stockings stood locked in the closet with my fur coats. Every now and then, I unlocked the closet to add something new to the stockings, followed usually by Polar, who did her best to get locked in. I would pass the closet later in the day to hear a muffled meow and I'd rescue her. Polar seemed to think something important was going on in there and she wanted to be a part of it.

While Charlie and John played pool, Placido Domingo's voice soared out Christmas music in the sitting room. Sandra and I ran upstairs to my dressing room to outfit her in some of my ball gowns and cocktail and dinner dresses. I sat on the end of my bed, my short, funky crew cut sometimes standing on end as I ran my fingers through it, my woolly socks sticking out from under my robe. I looked a bit like a waif who had no right to be there while Sandra slipped into my beautiful, big, kelly green taffeta ball gown and my emerald necklace and emerald clips. Sandra looked wonderful. We rushed her downstairs to show John and then took a photograph in front of the Christmas tree. Sandra was my Barbie doll this evening. It was almost as satisfying to watch Sandra in my clothes as it had once been wearing them myself. The dressing room was soon a flurry of silks, chiffons and taffetas. Designer originals were pulled out of closets and duly photographed on Sandra in front of the Christmas tree. It was such a good time.

Lindsay, Courtenay, Zuleika and Katrina now got into the act. Lindsay and Courtenay loved seeing their mother dressed up. I gave Sandra four dresses we thought looked best on her to take home to wear for a while. I told her, "Wear them and enjoy them at least until my hair grows in. I certainly won't be wearing them for a while." The crew cut simply didn't go with some of those floaty, feminine silks and chiffons. Should I accept any formal invitations, I'd wear my tailored black Yves St. Laurent dinner suit with the tuxedo trousers and jacket.

Soon it was bedtime for the girls, all camping in Zuleika's room in sleeping bags, where they giggled, talked and laughed until one in the morning. John was concerned that they were staying up too late, but I knew there was nothing we could do about it. Excitement was mounting in the house. Tomorrow night was Christmas Eve.

That night I slept in the dressing room again. My damned cold was worse. Christmas Eve Day I spent mostly in bed while John and Sandra bustled around doing — could it be possible? — more shopping. Charlie left "to pick some things up," as he said. By evening I felt well enough to go downstairs for dinner.

Jason had had a fight with his girlfriend and was depressed, which made me unhappy. He had bought her a beautiful Christmas gift, a black cashmere jacket, which he could ill afford, and now she didn't even want to see him or accept the gift.

Poor Jason. When he fell, he really fell. Ever since he was a little boy, Jason could be extraordinarily passionate in relationships, very much the one-woman man. I remembered a time long ago when we were all in Turkey while Charlie made *Dubious Patriots,* a movie with Tony Curtis, the title of which was later changed to *You Can't Win Them All.* Jason, at the age of seven, got a big crush on Tony's wife, Leslie. He wanted some private time with her, so he picked an old scab off his knee, making the old wound bleed, and went knocking on her door. He told her he had just fallen down and needed attention. Leslie picked him up tenderly, bathed his knee and fed him cookies. He was loyal to Leslie until he met the tall, attractive six-foot actress Jo Ann Pflug. He fell for her at eight and made her peanut butter and jelly sandwiches. Jo Ann called him her boyfriend and took walks with him. It was a sweet sight, the tall, beautiful brunette and the small, wiry little boy hand in hand. Jason was always lovable. I hated to see him sad.

But he was amused this night by Valentine, who was in a clownish mood. He danced around the sitting room, keeping us in stitches. Paul was there, also in a happy Christmas mood. I had a special gift for Paul, a pre-Christmas thank you for everything he had done. I had written a card saying how the last six months had been many things — terrifying, enlightening, frustrating and painful. But throughout that time there was one constant, someone I could always rely on, and that was Paul. I always knew he would be there for me, and I wanted to thank him. I had bought him a heavy, hand-beaten gold chain (a *keeper*, as my brother called it), something he could always keep. I gave it to Paul with my love and thanks. He put it on immediately.

Tony came by looking handsome in a dark suit. He was going to midnight mass and asked if anyone wanted to join him. I volunteered Sandra. I said, rather wickedly, "Sandra, would you like to go?" She had wanted to go last year in Vermont.

"Well, I would at any other time, but . . ."

"Any other time wouldn't be the same, Sandra. You wanted to go to Christmas mass."

"Well . . ."

I could see she was comfortable sitting on the floor sipping wine, and I laughed. "You don't have to go." She somehow slid out of the situation and Tony went with his friend Gary.

I teased Sandra after they left. "Last year you wanted to go to mass and it was twenty below freezing. This year you had the perfect opportunity. The weather outside is balmy. Tony would have taken you."

She laughed. "I know. That's just the way I am."

Pavarotti was singing. What a wonderful voice the man has. I loved Christmas Eve. The Christmas lights were twinkling. Everything was so nice. True, I was a little weak from the cold beads of perspiration formed in my eyebrows and I was giddy, but I was also happy. Soon the girls trooped in to say good night. Like all children on Christmas Eve, there was no trouble getting them to bed. Once more, the sleeping bags were piled in Zuleika's room.

The girls hung their small stockings in the fireplace, and Sandra and I filled them with a few small things: pencil sharpeners, erasers, pencils, candy canes and a China doll each. We attached the small stockings to the outside of the large ones. They looked wonderful. I was now full of excitement myself. Because of my bad cold, I slept in the dressing room once more. I didn't want to sleep by myself on Christmas Eve, but I couldn't risk Charlie's catching my cold. With the forthcoming ski trip one of the highlights of the Christmas agenda, I couldn't take chances. My cold didn't seem to be getting better. The family anxiously asked how I was doing and I said, "Fine, I'm feeling better." However, I was weak and the cold was not budging. I thought to myself, "It's happened again." I guessed I'd have to wait a bit longer before I started trying to glue myself back together again physically by exercising. We wished each other Merry Christmas and went to bed.

I was so excited, I was like a child. I found it difficult to fall asleep. I was also chilled and a bit trembly from the cold. I sat in bed thinking over the things I'd chosen and how everyone would like them. I couldn't wait for Christmas morning to watch my family open their gifts. I had left until this last minute wrapping Charlie's presents. I had been saving the most Christmasy wrapping paper for Charlie's gift. It was red with green holly on it and on each package I put a big red bow and a silver bell. I happily wrapped the Pavarotti tapes, the fancy long shoehorn, a teal blue cashmere sweater and a special Indian medicine bag full of different-colored quartz crystals. His big present was a pair of new Head Gold skis. I tied a big red bow on these and crept downstairs to put them under the tree.

I had been more relaxed about shopping this year but I seemed to have done as much as ever. I fell asleep about two o'clock and woke again at four-thirty, wide awake, remembering there was a gift I still hadn't wrapped — a piece of jewelry for Suzanne. It was still in my jewelry box. I found the last of the wrapping paper, tape, ribbon and a gift tag. Then I went downstairs and put it under the tree. All the family was asleep. The house was cold and I didn't linger. I got back into my warm bed with Polar and was soon asleep.

40

CHRISTMAS DAY.

The sound of the children galloping through the house and down the stairs awakened me. Immediately, I jumped out of bed, put on my robe and rushed downstairs. There they were, looking at their big, fat stockings.

"Oh, my God, Mom," said Zuleika, "they're so big. It must have taken so much trouble to do them. Oh, my God, Mom." They were all excited and couldn't wait to start.

I told them, "Let me wash my face and get a cup of tea. Then we'll all sit down and you can start."

Soon we were all assembled. Two sets of parents and four children. We were going to watch them open their stockings before the rest of the family arrived.

The girls had a routine. They sat down, took one thing out at a time and watched one another open each gift. It was time-consuming but they appreciated everything this way and I had the pleasure of seeing them open individually the gifts I'd painstakingly wrapped and put in their stockings. They loved everything. John took photographs of our daughters bedecking themselves with jewelry. Each girl was a colorful sight: Katrina, in a bright red angora hat and turquoise scarf, shiny earrings and necklace, was threatening to put on Day-Glo yellow socks; Courtenay had sparkly plastic bracelets up to her elbow; Zuleika donned black lace gloves with a glittery necklace and earrings; Lindsay draped a gaily striped shawl around her shoulders, a ski hat on her head and a jeweled necklace to match her glittery earrings and bracelet. They all munched chocolate candy. I studied Charlie's face. He wore the most wonderfully gentle smile as he took in the feminine scene. At one point I turned around and spied on a couch in the corner of the room a small green stocking. "Oh, look, Charlie, there's another stocking over there."

"Who's it for?" he asked.

"I don't know, but there's a card in it."

The card read: "For Jill."

"It's for me," I said. "There's a stocking for me!"

"Who's it from?" everyone wanted to know. I opened the card.

In print it read: *An old-fashioned Christmas tree wish — May your tree be evergreen, may your Christmas be ever glad, may your joys be everlasting*

Then written in pen: "And may you always be mine. I love you, Jill — Charlie."

It was a green silk stocking with a red cuff at the top, red velvet ribbon, bells and a pine cone ornament hanging from gold silk. It was a beautiful stocking.

I took it and hugged it. "I'm going to open this later. I want to keep it as long as possible. It's so beautiful."

The rest of the family trooped in. Suzanne arrived, followed by Tony, Paul, Jason and Valentine. Sweet, generous Suzanne arrived with an unexpected guest, her music teacher. Suzanne learned she would be spending Christmas alone, so she simply brought her along to join our family celebration. Tony and I each secretly pitched in one of our gifts so Suzanne's friend would not be empty-handed this Christmas. Everyone sat down to wait for the adult gift-opening to begin. I could see it would be a lengthy project. We all had placed gifts under the tree for days. It was a beautiful sight. Under and around the tree, our large family had piled presents high, one on top of the other, massing out into the room. The gift-opening was conducted in an organized fashion: Charlie gave them to Courtenay and she passed them to the recipients.

I sat on the couch with my stocking, taking it all in. It was difficult with so many people in the room, so many gifts being opened simultaneously. Boxes, wrappings, bows and ribbons piled up around me. My goodness, I was getting so many things this Christmas. And, oh my, so many from Charlie.

Charlie was like Santa Claus himself. He didn't sit or open his gifts. He continued handing out presents, which was quite a job. The kids urged me, "Open something, Mom." "Come on, Mom, open mine."

Everybody had been so thoughtful. People in Vermont had sent gifts. I was moved. Little touches of Vermont in familiar wrapping paper — a Zuleika Farm windsock from one of the girls who worked with the horses there, in our colors of camel and blue; a white nylon jacket for jogging from my friend and stable manager, Jane Ashley. And, closer to home, a buttery-soft suede shirt from John and Sandra; Day-Glo sweaters in shocking pink and bright yellow from Zuleika and Katrina. The gifts kept coming: a white silk peignoir from Paul; an eccentrically attractive bracelet from Valentine in brightly colored stones with a parrot on it; from Jason a huge sweatshirt with large shoulder pads — the girls loved it, oohing and aahing. A Bible from Tony, a beautiful leather one with my name embossed on it. A pink sweater from Suzanne with a white kitten embroidered on the front. Dino, who had been our loyal, much-loved houseman for ten Christmases, gave me some holy water from Lourdes and a silk scarf. James, our cook, came hurrying in, looking like Santa Claus, with a bottle of Joy perfume for me. The gifts were all so thoughtful. I had been saving Charlie's for last.

He gave me three good novels, big and fat. James had given me Joy, so two of my senses were satisfied. Then I opened my box of chocolates from Charlie — a nice big box of Godivas. Oh, wonderful, how marvelous. I opened a particularly big box to find a large rose-quartz ball. It was from Charlie. I held it in my hands. It felt wonderful, a very loving, warm energy. I started slowly on my stocking, savoring the moment. It was full to bursting, a cornucopia of feminine treasures: beaded earrings, a dear little doll with white furry hair and a tail — a little lion doll. It reminded me of the doll Zuleika had given me for my birthday the previous year, the one I took to the hospital with me and kept on my pillow throughout the ordeal. I pulled more magical things from my stocking: a small, clear crystal egg, as clear as my mind was on my last visit to Sue Colin; a small rose-quartz egg; then, at the toe, a little black box. I opened it.

"What's that?" I cried. It was a square-cut emerald ring surrounded by diamonds. "Oh, my God, Charlie, what have you done? It's so beautiful." I was shocked at the extravagant present. A perfect fit. Charlie had spoiled me. Everyone had spoiled me. I felt so loved.

Charlie opened his gifts. He loved his cashmere sweater, saying it was the perfect color for his blue jeans. He laughed at his medicine bag, emptying out the many different-colored stones into his palm, and declared the shoehorn just what he needed. He seemed happy and content. Then I gave him his skis, which I had hidden behind the sitting room drapes. He seemed genuinely excited by his skis.

His card, "And may you always be mine," told me eloquently that perhaps his best Christmas present was the fact that I was here with him.

Friends arrived: Sue Overholt, Kathy, King and Marcia. More gifts were exchanged and soon we all adjourned to the dining room for the feast. Our first Christmas dinner in Bel Air in ten years, and our last. It was a wonderful Christmas. I had deep stirrings of gratitude. Thank God I'd gone to Mitchell Karlan and he had found that lump in time. I was fortunate to share Christmas with my family and friends. For the rest of the day, the disease was far from my mind. I felt whole and happy.

With thoughts of cancer slipping farther and farther into the distance, I could hardly believe I had been ill. I felt as if it had never happened. Was this a healthy state of mind? Feeling as if I'd never been ill? As if I never would be again? It was as if I were washed clean of the disease and any thoughts of it. Even intellectually, I couldn't imagine having cancer. Well, maybe this was my most special Christmas gift.

After dinner, we were exhausted. We sat around talking, enjoying ourselves and our gifts and eating much too much. Later, once again we all exchanged happy Christmas thoughts and thanks and went to bed. I held Charlie tight. I was hoarse and losing my voice but I managed to thank him for his gifts, for the ring and the stocking and all that he had so thoughtfully put together for me to make this Christmas such a special one. Before getting into bed, I tied my Christmas stocking to the head of the bed, putting my little doll in the top.

Christmas 1984 had come and gone. What a year, one I would certainly never forget. It had given me an even deeper, richer appreciation of my life. Everything seemed unbearably lovely. I didn't want to give any of it up, not for a long time. I gave my nose one last hearty blow, reached up and caressed my stocking, feeling the silk and jingling the bells, and then I drifted off into a deep, sweet, dreamless sleep.

41

THE DAY AFTER CHRISTMAS, or as we call it in England, Boxing Day, Sandra and John went shopping to take advantage of Christmas sales. Charlie and I took one last inspection of the new house before closing the deal. I was happy in the house. It was beautiful and, for the first time, Charlie relaxed and enjoyed himself. He actually smiled at the prospect of moving in. We planned where to put our desks and where the paintings would fit. I wore my big green emerald ring, and everything felt new and special and very day-after-Christmasy. The house and the area around it were perfect. *Everything* was perfect. It scared me. It seemed I had never in my whole life had a setup that was more perfect than this.

"I've got everything," I said to myself. I looked at my new emerald ring. How old the stone was. It had been here much longer than I and it would be here long after I go. It made me anxious. It was so beautiful that somehow it seemed to mock me, making me powerless.

I supposed my unease was only my own desire to live a long time and enjoy all the wonderful things life has to offer. At home, I felt secure and well, but out in the world — even if only to visit the new house — I became a little frightened. But I recovered on the drive home. It was just the vision of how wonderful life could be near the sea. I envisioned quiet and peaceful walks down country roads to the barn. I had an inkling of a life-style I would enjoy: simplicity, smaller home, fewer possessions, a way of life that would be perfect for Charlie and me. All I had to do now was get healthy and stay healthy so we could enjoy it.

Two days after Christmas my cold worsened. I was tired after sleeping badly. I took care of my correspondence in bed, then meditated, sending white blood cells to my throat, nose and eyes, which were particularly sore. I had neglected meditation during Christmas. I had to get back to my routine. I hoped, as I concentrated on the white blood cells flowing to my throat, that they would do the trick.

The day before we were to fly to Aspen my temperature was high. My voice was hoarse and I had a croupy cough. I called Ray Weston, who said, "Take your temperature, dear."

I told him it was almost one hundred. He said, "If it goes up any more today, I don't think you should get on that plane." He knew how determined I was to make the trip. The whole family, with the exception of Jason, was going. For Charlie and me it meant a great deal. This trip would make up in part for missing Vermont. I knew I was damned if I caught the plane and damned if I didn't. If I did go and was ill, I would be a burden to everyone. If I didn't go, they would worry and it would spoil their trip anyhow. I really wanted to be with them. I would be trying my wings for the first time since surgery. I had been terrified of flying while I was ill. But now I had the confidence to do it.

Charlie didn't want me to get out of bed, but I left the house to see Bernard. I explained I had such faith in Bernard that I wanted to get on the table and have him go over me with his electromagnetic shooter.

John's appointment was at twelve, mine at twelve-thirty. While one of us received Bernard's personal attention, the other could lie on the table.

I asked Bernard how my brother was doing. He said John was in bad shape. He had been operating at only thirty percent of capacity; after five treatments, he was up to fifty percent. He reminded me to send our bottles of electrically charged water with the luggage and not to carry them in hand baggage. Bernard said the X-ray machines would cancel the electrical charge. He suggested John change his life-style and try to cope with business stress without running down his health. He knew many big businessmen who didn't succumb to stress. As far as Bernard is concerned, there is no such thing as stress, only situations and how people react to them. One doesn't necessarily have to become stressed over bad news or mounting pressure. One must find a means of dealing with pressure without becoming stressed. I understood what he was talking about, but I knew John wouldn't. Bernard said if John didn't find a way to avoid stress his health would break down and he would suffer a major illness. He said, "It comes to this, whether he loves the power of his business more than his health."

Bernard didn't believe I had a virus. He thought my fever and cold symptoms came from my liver, that I had eaten something that made me ill. He told me to stop eating dairy products. He had warned me previously that I was allergic to milk and cheese, but he knew I'd been eating them recently.

"While you're sick, no dairy products, no starch and no sugar. Just spend the day drinking fresh juices." If I wanted fruit and vegetables, I should have them two hours apart and not mix them. A suitable diet for the day: upon rising, a big glass of water and perhaps fruit or a small glass of orange juice; then a couple of hours later or midmorning, carrot juice or a salad; and for dinner, perhaps fruit again. He said I probably shouldn't take the tetracycline because my liver had already been through enough chemotherapy drugs and the bombardment of chemicals administered during surgery. He wanted my liver back in good shape.

"Every time you take something like tetracycline there are side effects on your liver," he said, adding that if I spent a couple of days sticking to juice, steamed vegetables and salads, I would get well fast enough. Bernard ran his shooter up and down my body, concentrating on my liver, the top of my head and the base of my spine. His shooter was a gauze-covered object, about the size of two bricks, on the end of a wooden pole about two feet long. Bernard held the pole and I lay on his electromagnetic wave table while he operated the shooter. The minute he started, I became deeply relaxed. I smiled to myself as I wondered what my doctors would say if they could have witnessed this science-fiction-type scene. However, I gave myself up to the total experience and in half an hour I felt better. Then it was John's turn. I spent another half hour on the table curled up on my side. I covered myself with my cloak and fell asleep.

When I awakened, John and I took a stroll in the park with a grateful Cassie. I told John what Bernard had said about him. "John, I wish you could find a holistic therapist in Toronto to help you handle pressure."

John listened when I suggested a holistic therapist. Sandra had said she thought he would never go for such a thing, but I hoped he would. I love my brother; I wanted him to learn from my experience. I didn't want him to become catastrophically ill to learn for himself.

On the drive home I felt fine. I came into the house, drank a glass of carrot juice and began packing for Aspen. I was sure I'd be well enough to travel. However, within an hour I was sick. I took my temperature: 100.2. I got back into bed. It looked as if I wouldn't be going until Monday, New Year's Eve Day. I looked at the bottles containing Actifed, tetracycline and Ornade that Ray Weston had prescribed. Oh, what the hell, I thought, my liver can handle a little more. I popped in two tetracycline and an Actifed. I should probably have done it earlier in the day. I might be better now if I had. I still clung to everything. I believed Bernard was helping me, but I also had years of faith in Ray Weston and his tetracycline. It was the only antibiotic I could take. I was allergic to everything else. It was important that this cold didn't go deep into my chest and make necessary stronger antibiotics, which I couldn't handle.

Charlie was worried about me.

"Why don't you stay behind and come on Monday."

"I really want to go with you. Everybody's so excited, I feel left out."

"The children are excited because it's part of their Christmas vacation. Sandra's not too excited. She's terrified of going on the chair lift. She's volunteered to stay behind with you until you come up."

Poor Sandra, she was scared of heights. I had made a Freudian slip earlier that day and said to her, "Oh, don't worry about the scare lift — I mean chair lift."

However, I had decided to be stubborn. "I'm going," I said. "I'm going. Me and whatever is left of my flu, or my cold, or my bad liver or whatever it might be, are going to get up and go to Aspen. I'm going to spend New Year's Eve with my family. I want to look the New Year squarely in the eye from the top of a high mountain. This tacky old cold is dealing with me, Jill Ireland Bronson; I've tackled bigger problems than a cold. I'm going to meditate and then whatever is wrong with me better watch out."

I carefully set out my clothes for the following morning. Polar sat on the end of my bed watching owlishly. I set out my blue jeans, Vogel paddock boots, a pair of thick, gray woolly socks and a big chunky sweater. Everything was ready. I was off to Aspen in the morning.

283

42

THE NEXT DAY MY VOICE was gone. I could manage only a croak and a whisper. I was racked with coughing and a terrible headache. Charlie came in in the middle of a coughing and choking session.

I looked up from the sink over which I was bending. "I can go, Charlie. It's only my voice. The rest of me is feeling much better."

Charlie smiled kindly. "No, baby, you stay in bed and come up in a couple of days. It's all arranged. You've got a ticket for Monday. You can fly up then. You won't miss much, just a couple of days."

I thought how all my "muches" were adding up, but I could see the sense of it, so I croaked good-bye to all the family. The long black limousine followed by a big white van, filled with bags, skis and down coats, and all my family, pulled slowly out of the driveway. "Good-bye, good-bye, don't be crazy on the slopes. Good-bye, I'll see you Monday."

I went back into the quiet house, back up to the dressing room. Louis Vuitton luggage was in the middle of the floor with Polar sitting on top.

"Meow," she said, "glad to see you." I got back into bed. It felt nice, warm and cozy. God, I was tired. I would follow Bernard's directions and eat only vegetables and drink juices for the next few days. No dairy products, wheat, meat or sugar.

Still and all, I had so much to be grateful for. It was now two weeks and two days since my final chemo. Normally, I would be facing another one in five days. I couldn't quite get it into my head that it was over. Every time I thought so, I touched wood. I remember Bernard's saying I was much better in every way. He recalled the first time he saw me; I was so full of fear that if a fly settled on me, I was frightened. I had been terrified right down to my bones. Every little thing was a threat, a possible sneak attack on my life, but now it was better.

All I had to cope with today was a bad cold and laryngitis. My ears were ringing, so I felt insulated in a cocoon of cold. Dino brought me a pot of tea and some juice. I sat in bed listening to the house. I heard Jason on the stairs. He was talking to my cat. "Hi, Polar. How are you?" I tried to call him but my voice was gone. I phoned down to the kitchen and Dino put Jason on the line.

"Hello, who is this?"

"It's your Mummy, darling," I hissed.

"Oh, Mom, you didn't go?"

"No. I'm sick."

"It's a good thing I broke my hand and couldn't go. I'll spend some time with you. There's a great old Jack Benny movie on TV if you want to watch. If you like, I'll go down to Nate and Al's and get you some soup."

"Thank you, sweetheart, I love you."

I could tell I was going to be spoiled for the next couple of days, so I swallowed my disappointment and put all my energy into getting well enough to leave on Monday. I had all day Saturday and Sunday, enough time. I snuggled under the covers and thought about my white cells. "Come on, chaps, rally round the flag."

Next morning I woke up feeling better. It was a sunny day, so I sat in the garden for forty minutes. "I think the way I'm going," I said to Cassie, "I shall be on that plane tomorrow morning." I spent the afternoon listening to Vivaldi's *Four Seasons,* which lifted my spirits. I felt better every minute. I wondered if I could take the chance and wash my hair. Well, better not be too cocky. I'd see how I felt by bedtime.

The house was alive, vibrating with the sounds of Vivaldi. Polar picked up my good spirits. She scampered up and down the staircase and in and out of the sitting room. After three days resting with me she was full of piss and vinegar. I was so uplifted I danced around the house to the strains of violins, singing, "Dum, dum, dum, di, de, dum; dum, dum, dum, di, de-de." Spring! proclaimed Vivaldi. Well, I did feel springlike. I felt terrific. I was definitely getting on that plane tomorrow. "Yippee! Look out, cat, that's my space." I danced around. Finally, out of breath, I sank down on the couch and looked at the Christmas tree for one last time. I knew when I returned from Aspen, Antonio would have taken it down. All the ornaments would be packed away for another year. I breathed the pine aroma. I remembered how much trouble Charlie had taken trimming the tree. I was enjoying dancing around it in my nightgown and slippers like a little girl on Christmas Eve, except it was the day before New Year's Eve.

Ray called. His voice was tired. "How are you today, dear?"

"Oh, Ray, I'm so much better. I think I can go tomorrow. I feel just great. I'm listening to Vivaldi."

"I'm so glad, dear."

"How are you, Ray? You sound so tired."

"Well, I was at the hospital all night. I had a patient of mine in surgery, but we saved his life, so it was worth it."

I felt a pang of guilt for feeling so good when my doctor was obviously worn out. "Take care of yourself, Ray, please. We all love you and we all need you so much." We wished each other a Happy New Year.

He told me, "Take a Sudafed first thing in the morning and then take an Actifed before you get on the plane."

I promised him I would.

I was more tired now. Too much dancing and prancing, I supposed. How marvelous that one high-spirited, redheaded Italian named Antonio Vivaldi still had the power so many,

many years after his death to uplift my spirits and make me feel whole. Life was full of so many wonderful goodies to enjoy. It was like walking through a magic cave with jewels embedded in its sides. Everything was there. All I had to do was reach out and touch. I would never live long enough to enjoy everything the world had to offer, but I was certainly going to try.

My New Year's resolution: to enjoy life to the fullest, all the sights and sounds, to fulfill all my senses. "Use it or lose it." I was going to play all my records, look at all the paintings, go to museums, enjoy the sunshine, enjoy the rain. I have so much; I am so lucky. My heart was bursting with gratitude. How wonderful to be alive. How wonderful to have the opportunity to live.

Polar careened into the room and stopped on a pillow, mad-eyed, tail all bushy.

"Piss off, Polar." Insulted, she dashed out of the room again, making me laugh heartily. She immediately returned and ran around the room. For one crazy moment I thought she was about to climb the Christmas tree.

"Don't you dare, Polar."

She scampered out of the room again. Dum-di-dum, dum-di-dum-dum, dum-di-dum-dum-dum-da-di-dum. Happy New Year, house. I was glad now I'd been sick and couldn't leave with the family.

New Year's Eve Day, I awoke early feeling much recovered, quite able to make the trip to Aspen. I dressed quickly, wished Polar Happy New Year and opened the windows to the balcony to shout to Cassie, "Happy New Year, Cassie. I love you." Then off I went.

Despite its being New Year's Eve, the freeway and airport were uncrowded. I arrived early and people-watched for thirty minutes. The atmosphere was light with happiness and bustling excitement. It was, after all, the last day of the old year. Obvious Christmas gifts were on display: new briefcases, sweaters, and I saw bright, sparkly earrings on several teenage girls, bringing to mind Zuleika, Katrina and my nieces. I boarded the plane to find it almost empty. It seemed everyone was already where they wanted to be for New Year's Eve.

Charlie had called the night before, telling me their first day's skiing had been pure chaos. Hordes of people were in the lift lines and it was standing room only in the restaurants and bedlam in the village of Snowmass. It sounded like a happy bedlam. The plane taxied down the runway. I didn't feel frightened or claustrophobic. I had come a long way. I could not possibly have flown anywhere in June or even August. I had been too full of fear then. I would have panicked the moment they closed the doors, locking me in with my monster. Now I felt like my old self, maybe better. The last time I flew had been on my way to Europe the previous February. I already had cancer, but I didn't know it. I only knew I was tired all the time. Standing at the airport had been an endurance test. Even simple tasks had taxed my limited strength. Yes, I was strong now. Maybe Alan was right. I was going to feel better than I'd felt for a long, long time. The huge drain on my strength was gone. It had been a trade-off in my favor; amputating my breast was not only going to save my life but give me a better quality of life. I fastened my seat belt. The plane made a smooth takeoff. I was on my way. Yea, me.

The lovely Christmas gifts notwithstanding, all I really wanted was health and strength, to be able to enjoy the physical activities that once gave me so much pleasure. I looked out the window, down on the snowcapped Sierra Nevada. I felt a surge of confidence and happiness. I stretched my legs. I believed cancer was far behind me. I was flying away from it. I was leaving it behind in 1984.

The cute flight attendant was attentive to his only passenger. He seemed to find me interesting, so I guess I looked whole and healthy, too. We flew over Boulder Dam and Lake Mead. Then I found myself looking down on the Grand Canyon with tears in my eyes. Oh, beautiful, bright, sparkling, majestic day. Fantastic. Thank you, God. Thank you for letting me see these things again. It's wonderful to be here on

Earth. I don't know what happens next, but it would have to be something to beat this. I was filled with joy, happy to be sitting alone. I could let the tears roll down my cheeks as I pressed my forehead against the window. I had never felt so completely alive.

We descended into Denver, floating down through white clouds. The sky was blue, and I noticed the moon, half-full, off to my right. We were running late. I would have to dash to catch the small commuter plane to Aspen. Denver was all brown — no snow. The plane landed smoothly and I set forth on my race through the airport, trying to pop my ears as I went. It was a long hike. The airport was under renovation. In and out of buildings, under temporary wooden tunnels and across runways. By the time I arrived, my left arm and shoulder were numb from my carry-on bag. It was probably the longest, and certainly the fastest, walk I had taken in a long time.

There were only a handful of people waiting to catch the plane, a very civilized group who looked as if they took this flight regularly. A blond girl in purple corduroy jeans and jacket and carrying ski boots sat beside me in the waiting room. Her heady perfume made me sneeze, clearing my sinuses and unblocking my ears. Apart from her, the other passengers did not look as if they were vacationing. They sat quietly and patiently. I wondered what they would all be doing at midnight. The blond obviously had plans; she tapped and flicked her long nails with her boarding pass impatiently. The plane was late now. After my marathon run, the wait was hot and stuffy. I told myself to let go. I relaxed and allowed my mind to wander.

I thought of Alan, how good he'd been. I hoped he was taking care of himself in New England.

My thoughts floated to Charlie, how impossibly difficult it had been for him to accept my illness. He denied its existence at times and went calmly about his life. At other times, his rage and frustration built to the point of explosion. Then we fought and tore at each other in a desperate need to alleviate the pain. For a man so accustomed to being in control and able to protect his family, Charlie must have felt impotent. He could only stand by stoically and watch me; but he did stand by me, sometimes just looking with helpless eyes while I thrashed, struggled and fought like a trapped wild animal. But eventually, through the long months and as my confidence grew, he had accepted my condition and found a way to live with it.

His most important gift was given me just before Christmas.

I had delivered a long speech: "Charlie, it's so awful sometimes. I feel so desperately afraid. I sit and think I'm not just scared of getting a cold or breaking a leg; this is big stuff. This is cancer. Where is it going to strike again? Thoughts of colostomies or losing my voice to throat cancer penetrate my mind against my will. I try not to think these thoughts and, Charlie, I'm trying so hard to build my confidence, to believe I will be well, truly well but, God, sometimes it's so hard. The other night after a perfectly wonderful day, I got up to go to the bathroom and it struck from out of nowhere — the fear, the reality — I've had cancer. I could get it again. I could die in a hospital, hooked up to machines, drowning in medication, pain, indignity and the awful hospital smells. Oh, God, I could be cut again. I didn't think all these thoughts one by one, Charlie. I've got it all down so pat; I can think and feel them simultaneously in one great big whump of fear. I even prayed last night, repeating over and over again, 'Please God, please God.' "

Charlie just held my hand silently, staying with me in the thought. He didn't try to escape in hearty words of encouragement or denial, he just stayed there with me. Then, after a while, as he felt it pass and I'd had enough space to feel and then move on, he said, "I expect it's worse at night," thereby giving me permission to feel this way around him and to express myself to him.

I replied, "Yes and no. It can come at any time just as bad, hit just as hard, but at night there are no distractions, so it's harder to shake. It's more isolated."

Then he said, "I love you, Jill." He accepted it all, and somehow I didn't feel so alone anymore. He had gone through the valley of fear with me quietly unprotesting, just walking beside me. It was a huge gift.

Living with someone going through as many changes and ups and downs as I did was undoubtedly hellish. It was an endurance test for Charlie; but he stuck to it, being there for me, a warm body, someone who loved me. While being totally supportive, he made me feel he didn't mind that I had only one breast.

"It's only a scar. It doesn't matter to me at all," he'd said. "As far as our relationship goes, it changes nothing."

I never doubted that.

Recently, since I was well, he seemed to show more concern for my health than he did throughout the time when things were very bad. He worried about my cold more openly than he ever seemed to worry about my cancer. Maybe only now he could allow himself to express any fear for me, and then only for something as curable as a cold.

I hoped Charlie was enjoying his skiing. I knew he needed the relaxation. I wanted to be well and whole for Charlie as well as for me, to regain my looks and vitality, to give him back his wife, to take away the sad look that I saw in his eyes when I caught him looking at me. I looked forward to seeing him. It was actually rather romantic, flying up the mountains to be together this way. I pulled out my compact and checked my makeup. Yes, everything seemed okay. I patted a little Opium on my wrists and in the small hollow of my throat and ran a comb through my hair. I was ready for 1985.

Finally, the plane arrived and we boarded. I climbed the metal steps of the gangway, dragging my coat and shoulder bag, giving the plane a friendly rap with my knuckles as I got to the door. I was excited and eager. We took off with a roar, shuddering and vibrating down the runway. It was a short flight, and in about thirty minutes we landed on the icy landing strip. Bump, slide right, bump, slide left. Then the roar of the engines as the pilot reversed the throttle, bringing us finally to a stop. I gathered my belongings and stepped out into the glare of white snow. It was cold, crisp, clean. The moisture in my nostrils froze as I walked across the tarmac into the small terminal.

I looked around. There he was, leaning against a post, wearing an old, familiar red down jacket, all ruddy from windburn and smiling such a happy smile. He was so obviously pleased to see me. Charlie kissed me, then folded me in his arms for a long while.

"You look good, baby, really good." It was as if we hadn't seen each other for a long, long time, and maybe we hadn't. After just two days, we came together with a clear, fresh new start. We looked at each other steadily.

"I made it, Charlie. I made it."

"You sure did. Happy New Year, baby."

"Happy New Year, Charlie."

EPILOGUE

May 1986
Los Angeles, California

Last month was my birthday and I looked back as one will do on such an occasion, not only on the last decade of my life but more significantly on the past two years.

Shortly after completing my chemotherapy, and having been told by my doctors to avoid stress at all costs, I watched my son Jason battle a two-month, life-threatening hepatitis from which, happily, he recovered.

I said good-bye to two friends. My brother-in-law Dempsey Buchinsky passed away unexpectedly from complications following surgery for a corneal implant, leaving all of us stunned and deeply saddened. My dear friend, ally and confidant Alan Marshall succumbed to Acquired Immune Deficiency Syndrome after a long and gallant fight. He is irreplaceable in my life.

I am sad to say that I never did meet my telephone friend Willie, with whom I had mutually comforting conversations. She also passed away.

I also lost my dog Friday, who died of cancer, and my sweet little friend Polar the cat, who had feline leukemia virus.

I had a more personal scare, in the grand tradition, some time ago. A new lump was detected in my left breast and a lumpectomy duly performed. I knew, though, following my inner belief and to my great relief, that it was not malignant. I followed the surgery with a five-week attack of bronchial pneumonia and a severe viral infection in my left ear. And then those threatening illnesses were behind me.

In spite of all, I have flourished like a weed. I haven't had reconstructive surgery — I no longer miss my right breast. In 1985, I co-produced the motion picture *Murphy's Law*, and now in 1986 I am currently enjoying co-starring with Charlie in a film in which I play the first lady, the President's wife. Charlie plays a secret service man.

Ever grateful to the summer of '84, I have learned that it's possible to survive great stress. The important thing is how you handle it. I know now that that is what counts most.

Surrounded by my family and good friends, I cherish my life, always mindful not to let my guard down. The fight must be continued.

J.I.